SURVIVING WOLVES AT THE DOOR

MY JOURNEY THROUGH CANCER

DWAYNE AND BARBARA MOORE

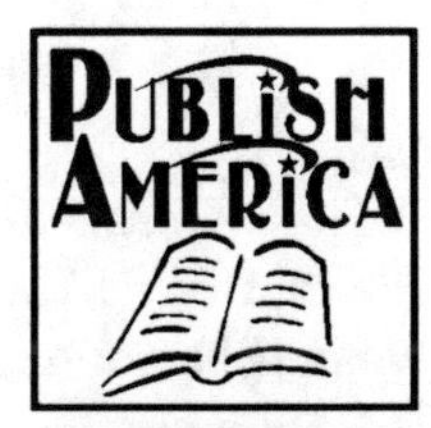

PublishAmerica
Baltimore

First printing

PublishAmerica has allowed this work to remain exactly as the author intended, verbatim, without editorial input.

ISBN: 1-60610-846-8
PUBLISHED BY PUBLISHAMERICA, LLLP
www.publishamerica.com
Baltimore

Printed in the United States of America

DEDICATION

This story, my battle with cancer and the impact that it has had on my life and that of my family is dedicated to the staff at the University of Virginia Cancer Center, the staff of the ENT Clinic, members of Second Wind, the wonderful people who work with NCCS, all of the friends who stood by us and helped us through this difficult time, and to my family: My mother Lorene, my sisters Darlene and Linda, my brothers Michael and Steve, and my extended family, and to my wife, Barbara without whom this effort wouldn't have been possible.

Most of all it's dedicated to my fellow survivors: who like me, refused to give up the fight, and continued to move forward one baby step at a time, wading through pain, stress, aggravation and all of the feelings that seemed magnified at the time.

PRAISE GOD that He brought us through.

If He takes you to it, He'll see you through it, and He brought us through for a purpose. Let's use this new lease on life to the best of our ability and to help those coming after us down this long and winding road of the journey.

Dwayne

FOREWORD

My wife and I met in early spring of 1998. We lived together for several years before we were married on October 28, 2001. During that time we had our share of tragedies to live through and put behind us.

Barbara was 5 ½ months pregnant with our daughter Faith, when, for medical reasons beyond her control, she miscarried. It was the hardest thing we had both ever had happen to us, and we felt like part of us had died with her. But with love for and faith in each other, we survived; becoming stronger people and our relationship only strengthened. Although physically she has been taken away, she is still with us in spirit and in our hearts today.

In June of 2000, we sat in the Hospice Unit at the University of Virginia Medical Center, as Barbara watched her mother slowly die as terminal emphysema shut down her vital organs. It was an emotionally traumatic experience for Barbara, because she and her mother had become so close after her dad's death in 1992.

We suffered the loss of our beloved Pastor Tommy in June of 2001, less than a year later. He had been a great friend to us both, and was like a father to Barbara—always there for her, through so many events of her life. She felt empty and lost without his presence.

In December of 2004, we tragically lost my nephew as the result of a horrific automobile accident. It deeply impacted not only Barbara and me, but the entire family and all of his friends as well. It is still something that we deal with every day. It was just another incident in a year that is one I wish could be forgotten

After dealing with so many tragedies and painful events in such a short time, we had every reason to believe that we could pick up the pieces and move on. Life would be full of laughter, and peace of mind, and of course the normal every day problems people are so used to dealing with that it is automatic and not something that we give a great deal of thought to. We could look forward to dealing with the every day life and growing old together.

Little did we know that only three short year's later, tragedy would once again come knocking at our door—and that it would change our lives forever.

Introduction

My name is Dwayne Moore. I grew up in Fluvanna County, Virginia—in the Palmyra district, a farming region in Central part of the state.

My mother and father both worked for a textile plant, and they worked what is known as the "graveyard" shift. Being the oldest of five siblings, it was my responsibility to look out for my younger brothers and sisters. Well—we all know about sibling rivalry, right?

Like most boys, I was active in sports. I played both little league and semi-pro baseball as a kid, and was a right tackle on both offense and defense of the Varsity football team.

I worked after school and on weekends baling staves for a lumber yard owner in the community.

I lived in Richmond, Virginia for a while and worked for an underground Utility Construction Company; and as an apprentice glazier when the Richmond Coliseum was being built, installing glass into metal frames. I eventually moved back to Fluvanna County.

Growing up and as an adult, I had health problems like everyone else. I would eventually get over whatever illness I had, returning to normal and going on without ever missing too many beats in the march through life. Colds and the flu went away and broken bones eventually mended—and life, in general was good.

In 2004, when Cancer—the awful "C" word, reared its ugly head, life as I had known it was brought to an abrupt, screeching halt. Sheer panic, disbelief, shock, being totally numb as the world spun crazily on its axle—unless you've been there and experienced it, there's no way to accurately describe what feelings and thoughts run over you and through your mind when you hear those words. Eventually, anger sets in—at yourself, those around you, and often times some even question God—how could HE allow this to happen to them? I never once questioned my faith, because without it, I would have been doomed from the start.

My whole life changed—and it was all because of that one little six letter word. My body was invaded by an unwelcome guest, my finances hit rock bottom, my weight plummeted like a stone thrown into water, food became a chore—a tasteless, bland unappealing struggle. What could I do? Where would I find the strength? Was there help out there to see me through? This is the story of the many different and often difficult choices I had to make, painful long treatments I had to endure, and the courage, stamina and determination I had to dig down deep to find to make it through.

God Bless,

Melvin Dwayne Moore, survivor

Barboursville, Virginia

DEVASTATING DIAGNOSIS

Cancer—it is the one word in any language that can strike the fear of God into the hearts, minds and souls of those who are diagnosed with it. Over the years I have known many people who have battled the disease. Some defeated it and recovered, while others lost their courageous fight and died. Most often it was because of a late diagnosis, or the treatments failed because of the type or stage of the cancer. Often, cancer is silent and doesn't present symptoms until it has grown or been present for quite some time, which makes treatment and or removal more complicated.

One thing I have learned from reading about cancer is we all have the cancer gene in our bodies. Sometimes they will mutate and become active, while others lie dormant for the person's lifetime. One of the people I knew who died from breast cancer was my paternal aunt, Alice. While I felt sympathy and compassion for them and the families they left behind, I felt like I was invincible.

Things like that happened to other people. I was a man who was strong, healthy, and full of vitality. I was totally in control of my life and nothing like that would ever happen to me. Life certainly has a way to throw curves when you least expect them, and to bring you back to earth in a jarring, teeth-shattering landing when you think you're untouchable.

My whole life was completely turned upside down on January 24, 2004. I was diagnosed with Metastatic Squamous neck cancer with unknown (or occult) primary, stage 2.

Several months earlier, I found a knot in my throat that was about the size of a quarter. It felt like small winged butterflies fluttering around searching for a place to land. It was a weird tickling inside of my throat, causing me to constantly clear it with an "ahem" here and another one there. Having to do that constantly was a little aggravating, but it wasn't something I was overly concerned about at the time.

My wife, mother and sister kept telling me I should have it checked by a doctor, but stubborn man that I am, I thought it was just a little minor infection or some kind of drainage from my sinuses that always plaque me, so I just kept going about my daily routine and ignored it. I've never been overly fond of doctors prodding and poking around, and would go only when absolutely necessary. I had awakened early this morning, and was ready for the day ahead. As I lay in bed stretching and letting my eyes focus and the sleep clear from my eyes, I thought of visiting my mom and brother for a while and then picking up some beer and snacks and settling in for an early evening of movies on television. Slipping quietly out of bed so I wouldn't wake my wife, I went into the bathroom.

Shortly after getting out of the shower, I noticed the tickling feeling had been replaced with more of a choking sensation. It felt like something the size of a golf ball had become lodged in the center of my throat. I noticed I was having more difficulty swallowing past it than usual; and my breathing was heavier than normal. It wasn't exactly painful, but was uncomfortable; it took a few extra gulps to swallow, and my throat felt full, like I couldn't get it all the way down.

I knew something serious was going on, and that the possibility of ignoring it for another day wasn't an option now. I was very scared as I stood in front of the mirror, because my breathing was more labored than it had been the night before. Thinking that it could be because I was almost in the panic mode, I tried to slow my breathing down, and began taking slow deep breaths, but it offered no relief. As I came into the bedroom to get dressed, I told my wife Barbara that I was going to go to the emergency room and have it checked out. She quickly offered to grab a quick shower and go with me, and as much as I appreciated her offer, I didn't see the point in both of us going. Assuring her that I would be ok, I dressed and went into the kitchen to make a pot of coffee before leaving the house.

Hospitals and doctors in general have never been a favorite place for either one of us, given our long history in dealing with them, and today was no exception. I thought it was some type of infection I had picked up from somewhere, so Barbara had agreed to stay home and do work on the computer that she had been postponing all week, before starting our Sunday dinner early. We would usually spend the afternoons relaxing in front of the television, or Barbara would talk with friends on the telephone.

We usually tried to drive down to Fluvanna County to visit with my mother and brother, but it would depend on how we felt after we ate dinner. Steve usually spent the afternoon sleeping and resting for the long work week since he got up early every morning, and mom would read for a few hours or find a good cooking show on television to watch. As I left the house, Barbara was beginning to peel vegetables for a pot of homemade vegetable soup to go with grilled cheese sandwiches. It was one of our favorite foods during the cold winter months, and it would save time cooking each day, as well as money on the grocery bill because we could have it for several days, and then put the rest into serving size containers and freezing them for another time.

It was a clear, crisp winter morning with the sun coming up, and a gentle brisk little breeze blowing as I walked out of the house. The trees on the mountain behind the trailer looked pristine as they waited for the arrival of spring to fill their bare branches with lush green leaves once again. So far, we'd been lucky and not had a hard winter like years past, and I was definitely looking forward to spring. I didn't particularly care for cold weather because arthritis had set into the joints and bones in different places in my body from old injuries years ago, and nothing seemed to alleviate the pain brought on by cold weather. Today promised to be another beautiful day and was indeed welcome. The forecasters had been right on the money when they had predicted a milder than usual winter.

During the 17 mile drive into town, traffic was lighter than usual for Sunday morning, and for once all of the traffic lights seemed to be in my favor as I whisked through intersection after intersection without having to sit in traffic. I wondered what the doctors would find when they examined my throat. What kind of infection causes all of the symptoms I had been experiencing lately? What medication was available to clear it up quickly without harsh side effects? I was sure they would be able to give me something that would soon have me feeling like my old self again, and that would be the end of it. I didn't particularly want to visit the Emergency Room, but on a Sunday, well, it was the only place to go and I didn't want to wait until Monday. The family medicine clinic where primary care physicians had their offices were always difficult to get an appointment with, and walk-ins were frowned upon now unless you called ahead a day. I didn't want to wait to get medication; and figured that the sooner I got it in my system the better.

When I arrived at the emergency room, I wasn't surprised to find the waiting room filled almost to capacity. That was normal because it was very seldom that it was NOT this busy. I automatically pulled into the parking garage across from the entrance, and remember thinking that it was a safe thing to do because the security guards would only make me move the car sooner or later. With free parking in the garages on the weekends for people visiting patients, it was hard to find a parking spot, and I drove to the top of the building before finding a space close to the elevators. Taking the elevator down to the ground level, I made my way across the street and walked into the emergency room. The steady hum and buzz of people talking amongst themselves was enough to make my ears roar, and I sighed in frustration as I settled into one of the small, uncomfortable chairs. I knew that I was going to have a long wait, and now I regretted not taking time to eat breakfast before leaving the house.

About an hour later, after I had munched out on a pack of nabs and a ginger ale, to stave off hunger pangs, they finally called my name. The nurse in Triage asked the routine questions about name, age, date of birth, what had brought me in, and proceeded to take and record my vital signs, before she sent me back out to the waiting room. Oh, well at least I got that far I thought, as I picked up a magazine and began thumbing through the pages to help pass time.

By the time the nurse called me back to the examination room, I was antsy and very frustrated. I had grown tired of sitting in rubber cushioned chairs that were not in the least bit comfortable—especially for long periods of time. The nurse led me around gurneys and wheelchairs in the hallway, down by the nurse's station and made several twists and turns down several short hallways before finally stopping at one of the larger examination rooms that housed 4 beds for patients.

As soon as the curtain closed behind me, she opened a drawer in the built in cabinet and gave me one of the open-backed gowns everyone despises, telling me to strip and cover up with a sheet. That really frustrated me because why should I have to get undressed to have my throat examined? Sighing in suppressed anger and frustration, I began unbuttoning my shirt as she stepped out to allow me privacy. Several minutes passed and she came back in to ask what had brought me to the ER and began checking vitals again. When she had finished documenting the results on my chart, she walked out without saying another word, finally mumbling that the doctor would be in soon as she exited the room. As soon as she left the curtained cubicle, it was pulled back again to reveal a member of the IV team.

She was carrying her trusty little caddy of needles and other paraphernalia that meant one thing: blood draw! "Oh Lord, "I thought, Dracula's on the prowl for victims again. It didn't seem to matter what a person came into the emergency room for, they were always determined you would leave a sample of your blood behind, and I would be no exception. She stretched out the rubber banding, making it snap like a big rubber band before placing it around my arm.

She drew the band so tight, it felt as if it was cutting off my blood circulation. Watching as she reached for her supplies, I could have sworn she picked the biggest needle she had in that damn caddy, and pushed it none too gently into my vein. Ouch!!! Hey, I thought, don't rupture it, as I cast an aggravated glance her way. She ignored me—twisting one vial off to replace it with another, rapidly filling three before finally dislodging the needle from my vein. It was already showing bruising, and without a word, she vanished as quickly as she had arrived, deftly closing the curtain with one flick of her wrist.

As I lay on that hard and uncomfortable gurney in the enclosed cubicle I tried to close my eyes and relax. Yeah, right, in an Emergency Room? Hah! That was a really stupid thing to think I could do. The noise and commotion drifting in from the hallway made it impossible, and seemed to steadily increase as the minutes ticked slowly by.

There were sounds of rescue squad members bringing people in with many different problems, the overhead speaker system paging doctors or sounding off calls to station repeatedly; and the sound of rushing feet as nurses and orderlies bustled and rushed around, transporting patients from one area to another, one test or x-ray, continually moving about while constantly chattering and issuing orders to others.

After what seemed to me like hours but was probably no more than forty-five minutes at the most, from under the curtain I saw black shoes and pants legs! Finally, I thought—the doctor's here so hopefully I'll be back in my car and on my way home soon. Well, of course I would have to stop by CVS Pharmacy and fill the prescription for the antibiotic unless he would be wiling to give me a dose for Monday morning so I could have it filled it at the hospital pharmacy before the end of the day. I had financial screening there, and paid a nominal amount for each prescription and refill.

The doctor came in, shook my hand and introduced himself, although I cannot recall his name after this length of time. I do remember noticing on his name tag that he was a medical resident. Oh, Great, I thought. He's still in medical school and he's going to know what's wrong with me? He examined my ears and throat with his little light before feeling of my thyroid with hands that felt as if he'd dipped them into ice before coming to see me, causing me to shiver. Whew! That certainly woke me up and I was wishing I had a blanket and not just a thin white sheet over me. The blood had been sent off to the lab to be analyzed so that in the meantime he ordered multiple x-rays to see what was going on in my throat.

Once he had the results of the x-rays and blood work, he still wasn't satisfied with those results, and came in to tell me he was ordering an Endoscopy to get a look into my throat. OH! Ouch! I'd heard how painful they could be, but had never had one done—but I agreed because I did want to know what was going on. But, damn I thought—how much more is he going to put me through before he writes the prescription so I can get out of here? I thought he was being overly dramatic about the whole thing, blowing it all out of proportion. Well, I suppose still being a student could account for that. The nurse who had took me to the room came in to wheel me down to the Endoscopy Department and said that she would see me when I returned to the ER before leaving.

After the technician explained the procedure to me in detail, he numbed my throat with a local anesthetic, giving it a few minutes to work—all the while assembling the instruments he needed and assuring me I wouldn't feel anything other than a little pressure. Who did he think he was kidding? There was no way that anesthetic was going to work that well or that quick. Just pressure, huh? I didn't believe him for a second, inhaling deeply as I prepared for the worse.

I knew better, and sure enough, as he began to work the scope down my throat, the pain brought a bunch of tears to my eyes. I felt my gag reflex ready to kick in, and remember thinking, "uh ho, here we go." Just a little pressure huh, as I tried to block out the pain and wishing he'd hurry the damn thing up, and I know it wasn't that long, but it seemed to go on for an eternity as I lay there on that cold and impersonal table with him working over me. I tried to think of pleasant things like fishing on a warm summer afternoon, NASCAR racing, anything to take my mind away from the fact that he was pushing a lighted scope down my throat and watching the images on the television screen of his computer.

Somehow, I managed to keep from vomiting, and he finished the procedure pretty quickly. I lay there for over an hour, wondering how much longer I'd have to wait for the results to come back. When he finally came in the room, the look on his face said BAD NEWS. Thinking maybe it was my tonsils or a severe throat infection, I was totally unprepared for his diagnosis—throat cancer!

Cancer! WHOAH! Hold on a minute, there buddy. I'm too healthy and active to have cancer. You made a mistake somewhere along the line, didn't you? But it quickly became evident that he hadn't, because he repeated that awful "C "word quite a few times.

I was totally frustrated because even with the Endoscope, he couldn't determine if it was malignant or non-malignant, didn't know the exact location of the tumor, nor could he tell me what stage it was in. My mind seemed to have frozen after the word cancer. I lay there on that gurney, my mind racing a mile a minute and his voice sounding like he was far, far away. Why me? How can I have cancer? "Oh, God," I prayed," I need your help to get through this! How can this be happening to me? I've never had a really serious illness my whole life, God—why now? What had gone wrong?

I have been a hard worker all of my life, and held a variety of positions during my years of employment. I've worked in construction, warehouse, housekeeping, as a contract flagman for the Virginia Department of Transportation, and as a truck driver. I've always taken pride in being a self-sufficient and independent person. So what am I supposed to do now, huh, I thought. How the hell do I tell Barbara that I have cancer? How is my mother, in her mid-seventies going to take the news that her oldest son has such a devastating disease? How would I find the words to explain it to her? And I had heard stories of how bad treatments for cancer could be and how people literally "wasted" away taking them—would that be what would happen to me?

The doctor finished his talk by saying he would call and schedule an appointment for me in the ENT Clinic later in the week. I needed to undergo more advanced testing. I was discharged a little while later, and as I walked out of the doors, I was completely numb and shell-shocked.

I was totally unaware of my surroundings as I walked like a robot to my car in the parking garage. I didn't notice traffic, people walking by me or toward me, and as the elevator doors closed, automatically pushed the button to the floor where I parked. I sat there in the car for several minutes, my mind in a whirlwind as I tried to calm myself down enough to safely operate the vehicle. I drove home on automatic pilot but remember very little of the trip. My mind was numb. Me—the invincible man—I had cancer.

I pulled slowly into our driveway, parking in the usual spot at the end of the trailer, just sitting there with the motor running, as I dug down deep to find the courage and strength to walk up the path and go inside, bearing news that would shock and totally upset Barbara. I shook my head to clear it and got out of the truck, walking slowly toward the back door. As I put the key in the lock, I silently prayed for God to give me the strength and courage to explain this to Barbara and the rest of my family and friends. What had started out as a routine Sunday had suddenly turned dark and bleak, and my courage was shaky at best as I stepped into the doorway.

Barbara was talking with some of her online friends when I got home. She turned off the computer and came into the kitchen as I walked in the back door, wanting to know what the doctors said. What antibiotic had they given me? Did I get it filled yet? I went to the refrigerator, grabbed a beer and opened it, taking a long pull to wet my throat and to give me a few minutes to settle down before answering her questions. She sat there waiting patiently but expectantly for me to sit down and tell her about what the doctor had said.

It was the hardest thing I'd ever done. I sat down at the kitchen table, taking another drink from the can and wiping my mouth. I had to look her in the face and tell her that the knot wasn't any kind of infection but cancer—and that it was all I knew at this point. As I slowly told her everything the doctor said I could feel it finally sinking in. And then I looked over at her standing at the other end of that table. She was visibly trembling as she held onto the end of the table, and her face had turned chalk white.

As long as I live, I'll never be able forget the look of total shock on her face as she collapsed into the chair behind her, causing it to slide back quite a way since it had wheels. She sat there, holding her chin in the palm of her hand, staring out the kitchen window with tears streaming down her face. "Oh, my God, Dwayne, no—they can't mean it. Are they sure?" She burst into long deep sobs, and we held onto each other, both of us crying by now and hugging each other as if we were holding on for dear life. Except when she had lost our daughter Faith back in the summer of 1998, I cannot remember ever seeing her cry with such gut wrenching sobs, even when she lost her mother to Emphysema in June of 2000. As sad as that event was, it was anticipated for some time, while today, this news—totally out of the blue, had floored both of us with such a unexpected wallop, I wondered how the hell we would keep it together to get through it.

After several long minutes, I became afraid her asthma would flare up or that she would hyperventilate, and knew I had to get a grip on my emotions. We both needed to calm down. I took a long deep breath and reminded her firmly but gently that nothing had been written in stone, and that the doctor could have read the test wrong. There was a chance we would get a completely different diagnosis from the ENT Clinic.

We talked about telling my family, but decided there was no point in upsetting anyone else until we knew something more concrete to tell them. It would be bad enough if the doctor hadn't made a mistake. We didn't want to upset them only to find out that it had all been a gross mistake by an incompetent resident.

We were both too upset after hearing the news to do anything except sit around the house, talking and just holding each other. I couldn't drive to moms and sit there without her knowing that something was wrong, and if she had asked, I know that I would have blurted it out. Barbara and I spent a very long and nerve-wrecking weekend, worried and wondering what the outcome of those tests would reveal. How did they treat cancer of the throat? What would I have to go through?

Would I be able to work? Eat? Would I have to end up with a tracheotomy? I had no idea what would take place and that was as scary as hearing that I had cancer—fear of the unknown.

I remember reading about people who died shortly after getting diagnosed with cancer and that scared the hell out of me. Would the same thing happen to me now? What was the percentage of that happening? I had lost my dad in his 50's from a massive heart attack, and my mother and sisters and brothers had different ailments that they lived with, but cancer? I was too young to have it, or so I thought at the time.

It wasn't until much later as I learned more and more about cancer and the people that it affects, that it shocked me. Children, babies even were diagnosed with cancer, and facilities like St. Judes Research Hospital in Memphis, Tennessee were filled with those precious little kids fighting this horrific disease. I learned that cancer is definitely non-partisan.

It was hard to concentrate on anything all weekend, and eating was something we did automatically, never really tasting what we ate. We both tried to shut it out of our minds, but it was there, just under the surface as the clock ticked seconds off so slowly it seemed like the hand of the clock never moved. I just "knew" in the back of my mind that the doctor in the ER, a resident, had made a mistake—he wasn't experienced enough, wasn't an attending; he was just guessing—all of it ran rampant in my mind, which just wouldn't quit jumping from one thing to the other constantly, never letting me relax all weekend.

The doctor I was referred to was Dr. James Reibel, one of the top head and neck surgeons in the ENT Clinic. They had moved from Hospital West out onto Fontaine Avenue into a new complex. Boy, they moved clinics around so much; it was hard to remember where to go anymore. They used to be in the Hospital West, and even Barbara couldn't picture where they were now. She had spent a lot of time there as a child due to lots of inner ear infections.

Never having been out to the new complex, it took me a while to find the right building, and then look for a parking spot. After registering down on the main floor, I finally found the clinic and had to sit in the waiting room for a while. I was as jumpy and nervous as a long tailed cat in a room full of rocking chairs as I sat there. Part of me couldn't wait for him to tell me that it had all been a big misunderstanding and yet part of me dreaded what would happen if it hadn't been one. I was finally called back to an examination room by one of the nurses.

After completing a thorough examination, he confirmed the original diagnosis of cancer, but could not be more specific until after he performed a biopsy and it was analyzed and staged by a Pathologist. Well, so much for thinking the doctor in the emergency room didn't know what he was doing, I thought, as I heard Dr. Reibel, (a cancer surgeon) deliver his diagnosis. He said the results should be back in a few days, and he did not want to wait any longer to find out what we were dealing with, and he was scheduling the biopsy for Saturday, February 7, 2004.

My eyes widened when he said biopsy, shocked that I'd have to go through that. He said that it was the only way to determine where the cancer was located and by sending it off for testing, to find out what stage it was in so they knew what treatment protocol to use to treat it. He rushed to assure me that biopsies were routine and hundreds if not more were done at the University almost daily, and that I didn't have anything to worry about. He filled out and signed a couple of papers, and said that there were others that I needed to get done that day in order to get myself registered into the system for the biopsy.

My appointment with Dr. Reibel was early in the morning, and Barbara had been unable to go with me because she was having problems with her monthly cycle, and had severe cramping and back pains. The only relief she found was lying down. She was having more and more problems with her cycle each month, and we were both beginning to worry about it. Whenever she approached her gynecology doctors, they took the attitude that with her age it was routine and nothing to worry about. Well, they didn't go through it, and they weren't the ones too weak to get up and down, other than rushing to and from the bathroom constantly to change to prevent leakage.

I was confident that I wouldn't be gone very long, and promised to pick her up a burger and fries on my way home. I should have known better than that when dealing with clinics and hospitals. Between completing tons of paperwork because it was my first visit to the ENT clinic, and of course the usual wait time to see the doctor, it was late afternoon before Dr. Reibel sent me over to Pre Admissions in the main hospital. I had to fill out insurance papers and other forms before the biopsy that was less than a week away.

When I didn't come home, Barbara became very concerned after 4 O'clock in the afternoon. She called the ENT Clinic and was transferred from one place to the other, before she caught up with me in Pre Admissions. Shocked at where she found me, she bluntly asked "what the hell are you doing in Pre Admissions?"

I have no idea what ran through my mind at that moment or why I did it, but I blurted out "Don't fall apart until I get home, but I have throat cancer." DUH!!! How could I have been so damn stupid? Of course she was going to fall apart.

I think I was just so damn scared and upset, after learning that it was cancer and in order to find out how bad it was, meant that I had to have surgery, that I had to tell someone what I was dealing with and how I felt; and when I heard her voice on the phone, the dam that had been building inside me since he confirmed the cancer broke. It came out with a rush before I could think rationally. I felt like I was drowning and I needed someone to hold on to.

Barbara's Reaction to The News:

I couldn't believe what I was hearing! They actually confirmed that it was cancer? And he didn't want me to fall apart? Who was he kidding? Of course I fell apart, literally right there on the spot as great sobs engulfed me, threatening to overpower me right where I had collapsed onto the commode. Oh my God, he's going to die, I remember thinking. I had heard so many horrible stories about people who suffered and wasted away when they found out that they had cancer, and I couldn't believe that I would have to wait and see Dwayne punish like that. Cancer was a horrible disease, and my mind was in a whirlwind as one thought after another occurred to me, nonstop—until I actually felt dizzy. Radiation burned people, didn't it? What about cobalt? (I had no idea that those treatments had been discontinued over a decade prior to his diagnosis). How was I going to be able to take care of him at home without any help? Would he be bedridden and unable to care for himself at all? I was becoming quite panicked and weak from the images that my mind was conjuring up when from out of nowhere, I heard Tommy Lewis' voice saying, "Barbara, turn to God right now and call Sandy." Tommy, our former Pastor, had been a rock for me whenever I was faced with overwhelming problems and someone I could trust even with deep dark secrets that I hadn't shared with another living soul. I knew that Tommy was looking over me when I "heard" his voice. A feeling of complete calm and peace washed over me as I felt his presence there beside me, and I began taking deep cleansing breaths of air. It wasn't until then that it dawned on me that I had been taking such short shallow breaths; my lungs were actually burning from lack of oxygen, and I felt my head spinning.

Trying to get a grip on my ragged emotions, it took several tries with trembling fingers before I was able to dial Sandy's cell phone number, saying a silent prayer that this would be the one time that she would actually answer the phone and that her voice mail would not pick up, forcing me to leave a message. I was still having a hard time controlling my breathing and the tears were still steadily streaming down my face unchecked.

Sandy, with a busload of school children on their way home after a long day in the classroom, finally picked up the telephone, and knew instantly that something was wrong when I was barely able to do nothing more than whisper her name into the receiver. Taking a deep and shaky breath, I managed to tell Sandy what was wrong, and she immediately pulled the bus off of the highway and began praying for both Dwayne and myself. It was so quiet on the bus you could hear a pin drop, with no child making as much as a sound. As Sandy prayed, I felt like the weight of the world was lifted from my shoulders as I turned the entire matter over to God and asked him to take care of both of us according to his plan. Of course, after being on such an emotional rollercoaster, and hearing such devastating news over the telephone of all things, I wasn't able to completely calm down, and spent some time when I hung up crying and just "coming to terms" with the news. But I knew that I had to get control because it would make it that much harder on Dwayne to deal with if he saw that I was a complete basket case, because he would be more concerned about me than himself, and I couldn't allow that to happen.

Dwayne's View:

As soon as I hung up the phone, I cursed myself for being all kinds of a fool. Here I had told her I had cancer, and she was by herself miles away from me, when I couldn't reach out and comfort her or hold her. The hands on the clock moved at a snail's pace after that. The woman handling my paper work seemed to move in slow motion as she entered my information into her computer, asking question after question, frazzling my nerves even further. I worried for the rest of the afternoon. Was Barbara alright? Finally, in desperation I prayed, "Lord, please watch over her, until I get there."

By the time I got home, it was just after dark. Every light in the trailer was on. It was as if she turned on lights, it would keep at bay the darkness that must be threatening to overwhelm her. As I walked into the house, Barbara was visibly shaken, and sitting at the kitchen table, smoking a cigarette. She had fat tears streaming unnoticed down her cheeks, and a bad case of hiccups from crying. Walking to her, I got down on my knees in front of her chair; she wrapped both arms around me, burying her face in my shirt as she cried even harder.

I stroked her hair, trying to calm her down, until after a few minutes, she managed to regain a little control. I found out she called our Pastor, Sandy Kelso immediately after hanging up with me. Sandy, who at the time was a part-time bus driver for Albemarle County Schools, had pulled off to the side of the road, to pray for me and Barbara and for healing of the cancer in my body. At the time, the bus was loaded with kids, but my wife said it had been so quiet you could have heard a pin drop.

Sandy and Barbara had been through a lot together with Sandy's first husband Tommy. Tommy had been the Pastor of the church, until in bad health, he had to retire. He was diabetic and had degenerative heart disease and was often bed-ridden for days at a time. We have also been through a lot with each other since Barbara and I had been together. Sandy had been very shaken by the news. She is a very loving person and has a big compassionate heart.

We knew since the biopsy date had already been scheduled that it was time to pay a visit to my family and break the news to them in person. I dreaded this trip, more than I can put into words. I knew my brother could come to except it, but I was really worried about my mom. I had learned my lesson about using the telephone for something this important and shocking and I wanted to be there in person, to try to comfort them—or was it that I needed their comfort for myself?

My mother, Lorene and my brother Steve took it with surprisingly more calmness than either Barbara or I had anticipated. They did have a lot of questions to ask. Was it malignant? Had it spread? Would they use Chemotherapy or radiation? What did the doctor think the outcome would be? Other than being able to tell them the date of the biopsy, I really didn't have the answers to any of their questions. I had been so numb with shock and disbelief I had not known what to ask.

Looking back now, I really didn't know what to ask. I had never once thought about cancer as something that would touch the life of someone close to me and especially not me. It never dawned on me to ask someone who worked with the patients and their families if they had information packets or brochures that we could read to find out what to expect. It would be quite a while into my journey before I realized how many organizations, websites and other helpful information was available to those who had been diagnosed. All I could tell them was I would let them know when I had more news. It was with a heavy heart that Barbara and I left for the drive back home.

At church the following week, Sandy and the congregation prayed over me and Barbara, as the date of the biopsy moved closer and closer. As it approached, we were more nervous and anxious than we had been the day before. After the service, Sandy asked who was taking us to the hospital and offered to drive us in.

I would not be able to drive when I was released, and Barbara had trouble driving my truck, because it pulled the muscles in her back more than driving a car, and it didn't help that the truck didn't have tilt wheel either. Sandy said that she would pick us up and drive us in so we wouldn't have to worry about looking for anybody else.

Sandy picked us up at 6 a.m. Saturday morning, and her teen-age daughter Renee, was trying to snooze in the back of the van. We were quiet for the most part on the ride in, although we did talk a little, and Sandy prayed as she drove down the highway. As we got into town in the morning rush-hour traffic, Sandy almost caused all of us to have heart failure. At one of the busiest intersections in town, directly across from a major shopping center, she turned left on a red light that she should have yielded at, right in the path of an oncoming vehicle. I think my heart skipped about three or four beats, while Renee was yelling, "MOM"! At the top of her voice, directly behind me, causing my ears to buzz and roar like someone was ringing a bell in them.

Verifying the Verdict

When we arrived at the hospital, we went to the Admissions waiting room to check in. The staff in the operating room would come down to get me when it was time for the procedure. We were surprised to see my mother, my brother Steve, and my two step-children from a previous marriage, Tina and Wade waiting for us. They had not said anything about coming, but it was good to see all of them. I was a nervous wreck and my stomach felt as if a million butterflies had taken up residence, constantly churching and flipping. Because I would be put under anesthesia for the procedure, I had not been allowed to have anything to eat or drink after midnight, and I was hungry and thirsty. My hands were wet from sweating profusely, causing me to constantly wipe them on the legs of my jeans.

Sandy parked the van at the main entrance and walked with us to the Admissions waiting room, wanting to pray once more with us before I went upstairs. Saturdays were usually her day to pray and prepare the sermon for Sunday service and she said that she would go on to the church and would leave her cell phone on, and that we should call her when I had been discharged. She would come back and meet us again at the main entrance and stop anywhere we needed to before taking us home.

As soon as Sandy walked out of the door, the receptionist called me. It was time to go upstairs to the Operating Suite. Barbara, trying really hard not to cry, went with me. My stomach did somersaults as I began walking toward her, wondering what would lie ahead of me when I got upstairs.

It felt weird as the big doors of the operating suite opened to allow us to enter in. I had worked here as a housekeeper for almost two years, and there were several of the staff I'd worked with on duty as we were pushed to the cubicle I would occupy. Alice, behind the glass and who ran the intercom system for the operating area, waved at me and smiled. I tried to make a joke by saying I didn't think the next time I saw her it would be with me as the patient, but the joke fell flat. Even she didn't smile.

Barbara helped me get undressed and into the gown, booties and surgical cap. She folded my clothes and placed them under the gurney in the wire basket. We had to wait for Dr. Reibel's team to come by before I went into surgery. Each member of the team came into the little cubicle, introducing themselves and explaining what their job was. I remember thinking as each came in that it was sure a big team for such a simple procedure; which did nothing to calm my already jingly nerves.

One of the nurses, who had an attitude that said she had gotten up on the wrong side of the bed, was determined that I sign a paper giving them permission to do a blood transfusion, if it was needed while I was on the operating table, and kept saying I needed to sign and date it before they took me into surgery. Since Dr. Reibel had not mentioned this, I didn't want to sign it. Why should I need a blood transfusion anyway? Dr. Reibel said that it wasn't a complicated procedure and certainly not a really long one.

Finally exasperated by the nurse's attitude, Barbara sent her off to the operating room to ask Dr. Reibel if it were necessary. After about ten minutes, she returned. She picked up the paper, and ripping it in half tossed it into the trash can, before turning to strut out of the cubicle, tossing the curtain aside impatiently, causing it to swing for a while as it came back together. I glanced over at Barbara and quipped: "Well, I guess we put a crimp in her bonnet for the day," which caused her to smile a little. I was glad to see that smile no matter how small it had been.

Barbara and I spent the rest of the time before I went into surgery just holding hands and hugging each other. She pulled the uncomfortable looking wooden chair close to the bed, laying her head on my shoulder, as I put my arm around her shoulders. I was afraid to try to talk past the lump in my throat, not the one they would biopsy—but the one choking me from holding my emotions in check. But wanting to reassure her, I finally managed to speak—telling her that I would be ok, I was too stubborn to let a little thing like a biopsy put me down. "We'll be out of here and back home before you know it." Maybe I said it more to convince myself than I did to reassure her.

When the orderlies came to wheel me into the operating room, Barbara tried so hard not to let her tears fall. They slid down her cheeks as she took deep breaths to keep from falling apart. I didn't want my last glimpse of her to be of her crying so I gave her a kiss and thumbs up, not wanting her to read in my eyes how damn scared I was. The gurney began rolling toward the operating room with all those big lights, and so much of the unknown. She waited patiently for one of the nurses in the Operating Suite to get a few of her errands caught up. She would get a wheelchair to take her back downstairs. In the admissions waiting room, she rejoined the rest of the family. When she got there she told them the nurses said it would be about an hour procedure, and they would call when I was back in the recovery unit. Too nervous to sit still, she fidgeted and moved around in the chair until she couldn't take it anymore. Finally, she decided she just had to get some fresh air and headed for the door.

Barbara, Tina and Wade went to the cafeteria for some much needed coffee, and then outside to the enclosed smoking area. Barbara was probably ready to chew a cigarette instead of smoking it, because she was so nervous and upset. Tina, out of habit or because she was nervous, talked non-stop and the chatter nearly drove my mother crazy, causing her to get a severe headache.

The operating room was much bigger than I remembered as the orderlies wheeled me inside. Of course, back then when I was working here, I had always walked into the room with cleaning supplies. They wheeled me over beside the big operating table with the huge overhead lights. Taking a deep breath, I managed to scoot over onto the table and having one of the nurses' lay the cloth over me.

Once I was in place on the operating table, Dr. Reibel assured me that the surgery was a routine procedure and I would do just fine. I remember thinking to myself: "yeah, right. You're not the one laying here on this cold piece of steel, waiting for some guy with a funny cap on his head and a mask hiding his face, to slice your throat open with some funny little knife." Then the Anesthesiologist stepped up directly behind me and that was the last thing I remember. In order to find the exact location of the tumor, Dr. Reibel and his team performed a tonsillectomy, and they discovered the tumor lying behind my left tonsil.

I woke up in the recovery room a short time later, with my eyes having trouble focusing on anything around me. My mouth was so dry it felt as if I had swallowed a bucket of sand or chalk dust. The first word I managed to croak out was "water"—but was told I had to wait, because they needed to make sure I wasn't going to vomit before they could give me anything. I had a bad case of dry heaves, where I would retch; but with nothing in my stomach since early the evening before, there was nothing to come out. Thankfully, within a few minutes, I was able to get some ice chips down that soothed my parched throat. It was very painful to swallow, or so I thought. I had no idea that the pain would increase even more once the entire anesthesia had worn off, and before the pain medication he had given me could take affect.

As I was wheeled back into the little cubicle I started from, Barbara and my mother were there waiting for me. My wife, who can be stubborn when needed, had been insistent that they allow my mother to come upstairs with her, and the nurse hadn't refused. Between the two of them, they managed to get me dressed. I couldn't help much, as I was still woozy from the anesthesia and light headed. My fingers didn't want to cooperate no matter how hard I tried. Once my mother had seen for herself that I was alright, she left so Steve could drive her home. Barbara struggled through getting my socks and shoes on, and was breathless by the time she sank down into the wooden chair. We had to wait for someone from the transportation department to take me downstairs to the main entrance.

Barbara called Sandy at the church when we were ready, and she came back to pick us up. Since I was still feeling some of the anesthetic, we decided I would be more comfortable in the back, since it would recline if I wanted to nap on the drive home. She stopped at CVS

Pharmacy on Long Street to fill a prescription Dr. Reibel had written for pain medication, liquid Roxycet since it would be easier for me to swallow than in tablet form, and boxes of tissues that would be a must for me over the next few weeks.

When we got home, I was still very weak and disoriented from the anesthesia. Sandy helped Barbara walk me inside and to get settled into my recliner in the living room. I needed something to eat before taking any of the pain medication. I managed a light lunch of some fruit and ice cream and an Ensure. I gave into the need to lie down for a nap. I was asleep before my head was comfortable on the pillow, and slept for several hours. The pain wasn't so bad, and the medication Dr. Reibel prescribed worked rather quickly, although it did cause some bouts with nausea, especially if I didn't eat something before taking it. Applesauce and pudding was the only thing I could manage for a couple of days that didn't cause severe pain when I swallowed—and of course my favorite—Neapolitan ice cream.

With the biopsy now behind us, things should have been easy—I mean that was the hardest part to go through, right? NO! Now the really hard part began—waiting for the results of the biopsy to come back from Pathology. We had ten long, hard nail-biting days to get through. We talked about it so much we nearly drove ourselves and each other over the deep end. We kept saying: ok, we're not going to think the worse. In the back of our minds, we both did and were too chicken to admit it to each other. Finally, Dr. Reibel's office called and asked me to be in his office at 11 a.m. on February 17, 2004.

As I drove toward Fontaine Research Park, I said a silent prayer that if it be God's will, the results would be something He, Barbara and I could handle together—with Him in the lead and with us following His

Will. I tried to concentrate on the traffic and turned on the radio to listen to music, hoping it would help take my mind off what they would tell me when I got to the doctor's office. I love listening to country music and they played some of my favorite tunes on the drive in, including Alan Jackson.

When I arrived at the clinic, there were a few other patients still waiting to be seen but it was not as crowded as it had been on my first visit, for which I was thankful. I registered at the desk, and took up a magazine to occupy my time as I waited to be called.

As I sat there in the waiting room, my mind went into a spin. What had he found? Was it worse than he had thought? Would he have to do a tracheotomy? Would I lose my ability to speak? I tried to calm myself down. No use borrowing trouble where trouble doesn't exist I chided myself. Have a little patience. His nurse called me back to the examination room within minutes after as I was seated. We stopped by the step-on scale for the routine weight check. She took me into one of his examination rooms, where she checked my vital signs before putting my chart in the holder on the wall and closing the door. I was very fidgety sitting on that exam table, my mind racing over what I'd already been through, and wondering what he would tell me when he came in. "Lord," I prayed—please let it be something with at least some good news that we can handle together."

I didn't have to wait long before Dr. Reibel came into the room. I was unconsciously holding my breath as he opened my chart, reading the contents before speaking. He told me that the Pathologist, after examining and staging the tumor, found that it was non-malignant and at Stage two.

He explained it meant we had caught it early. It was measured to be about the size of a medium walnut. I let out a pretty audible sigh of relief. Cancer, yes it was; But it wasn't as bad as it could have been had I waited any longer before actually going in to be seen back in January. Life threatening and would likely spread to my other organs? NO. Praise God for answered prayers. It was the first time I think I had actually managed to take a deep breath since I had walked into the clinic. What a relief, and I felt 100% lighter. I knew there were probably still a lot of things I would have to deal with, but I wasn't facing a life threatening situation and that was reason enough to at least celebrate a little.

I shook Dr. Reibel's hand gratefully and enthusiastically at the news. Part of me couldn't wait to share the good news with Barbara. I wanted to see the look on her face when I gave her the news. I had learned my lesson and was not going to call her. I did not want to hear it in her voice on the other end of the telephone.

Dr. Reibel didn't want to postpone getting started with my treatments, and in order to start as rapidly as possible he gave me a referral to the Assistant Professor of Radiology/Oncology Dr. Paul Read. He would do his assessment and give me a detailed look at the treatment options available to me.

I was almost giddy with relief, and felt like I was floating as I drove home. I couldn't wait to share the good news with Barbara. We had been worried and stressed out since this nightmare had begun. I wanted to tell all of my family and friends that while it was still cancer, it was treatable and manageable. I would share this part with them first, since they were all waiting to find out what the doctors had found, and then once I knew more after seeing the Radiologist/Oncologist, I could fill them in on what he said.

Of course, there were tears again when I told Barbara the news—but unlike the last time, they were tears of relief and joy. I even shed a few of my own tears—who said grown men aren't supposed to cry? I felt like all of the tension that had been bottled up inside of me, finally broke free and I could at least relax for a while and enjoy this piece of good news. It was such a relief to know that yes, while it was still cancer and I would have to go through treatment, it wasn't life threatening or likely to spread to other organs, which was my main worry.

We knew that it would be a long journey, but we would manage somehow. We felt like we'd been granted a reprieve and from now on, we were just going to take it one day at a time and try not to panic at every bit of information we were told.

A few days later, I drove to my appointment with Dr. Read with more composure than when I had visited Dr. Reibel earlier. I had no idea what he would tell me as far as my treatment options were concerned. That part really didn't matter to me because I had made up my mind whatever he suggested was necessary I would do without question or complaint—well at least to a reasonable point, anyway. He was the trained professional who probably had dealt with more cases than even I could imagine. I had to trust him to know what would be the best way to handle my case.

Not being familiar with the West Complex of the Medical Center, I stopped at the receptionist desk to ask for directions. I was surprised it was easy to find, and it was on the main floor. Which meant—no elevator rides? I wasn't exactly claustrophobic—but, well—let's just say I preferred to stay on the outside of elevators looking in.

Dr. Read was a young doctor to have such a demanding, and senior position on the staff. He was very friendly and outgoing, and with his boyish good looks and charming personality, I could envision a lot of his female patients wanting to swoon at his feet. He wore a bright smile on his face as he entered the room. Gripping my hand in a friendly, firm handshake, he sat on the spinning stool at the foot of the exam table where I was seated. He had already read the notes on my case, but glanced over them briefly before doing his own personal examination.

Then, in simple every day language I could understand, he outlined the options he felt would be best suited to handle my case. He suggested that the best way to handle my particular case was with radiation therapy combined with an aggressive dose of chemotherapy. I agreed with his assessment and we set the radiation therapy at 5 times per week—with each treatment averaging around 20 minutes each, although sometimes they might go as much as half an hour, depending on the dosage being administered.

He said before I could take the first treatment, I would need to shave my beard and any hair on my neckline so it wouldn't interfere with the radiation. Uh ho—umm—shave my beard? But now, hey wait a second, I thought, I've always worn my beard since I had a steel plate surgically implanted for a broken jaw years before. Oh, well, if it meant beating this cancer, what was doing without facial hair for a while? I could always grow it back after I finished all of the treatments and whatever else I would go through. I didn't quite understand why I had to shave my beard off if the radiation was going to be concentrated on my neck and throat area, but who was I to argue if the treatments worked?

The other thing he explained was that I would have to be fitted for a special mask. It would go over my head during the radiation treatment. When they fitted me for it, they would use permanent markers to locate the precise area where each dosage of the radiation would be concentrated. He was very up front and honest, which I appreciated. He said I would probably call him every name in the book and a few more before it was all over, and it was going to be one hell of a ride, but to be cured I had to suck it up and take it.

He just struck me as a down to earth, ol' country boy type with his open friendly personality and I thought that he and I would get along just fine. He was very straightforward and didn't beat around the bush.

He gave me a referral to the Cancer Center to see Dr. Christopher Thomas, a Chemotherapy doctor, for his assessment and an explanation of what to expect from that part of the treatment. Whew, I thought! There are certainly enough doctors working on my case to beat either the cancer or wear me out trying. It seemed like it just wasn't going to be enough time in the day to fit all of these appointments in each week. I was beginning to understand that the only time I wouldn't be spending at the hospitals were going to be the weekends, when I'd probably have to spend time building up energy for the next go-round starting again on Monday.

When I first met Dr. Thomas in the Chemotherapy department I wasn't fond of his attitude and demeanor. He was a very gruff and "sour puss" type. Once again, I was put through an examination. He explained how the chemotherapy was administered. He would be prescribing an oral chemotherapy tablet I would take twice a day for 2 weeks and then stop for a week. I would be required to come into the clinic for blood work, and then every two weeks, would come in for IV infusion. He was hopeful that the combination of two chemotherapies would shrink the tumor to a minimal size that could be removed surgically, without causing a great deal of trauma.

The drugs were very expensive, and he suggested that I contact one of the social workers in the Cancer Center because they could help me apply for financial assistance that was available to those with no or limited income. One thing Dr. Thomas was adamant about before he started administering chemotherapy, was that I be scheduled to have a PEG (feeding tube) surgically inserted into my stomach. Feeding Tube??? Now, wait one minute. I can eat fine on my own, I assured him—I don't need to have a tube put in my stomach! He refused to budge—stubborn old man! He said I might feel like I didn't need the tube, but eventually I would experience problems eating as the treatments progressed. Uh, huh—sure I thought.

After the appointment, I asked at the receptionist desk how to get in touch with a Social Worker for Cancer Center. They asked me to have a seat in the waiting room and they would page a worker for me. I was surprised when the social worker arrived.

Vikki Bravo, (who it turned out was the Senior Social Worker of the Cancer Center) was what people in the country describe as "no bigger than a minute", very petite and short, with dark wavy black hair, and had what I would later come to describe as an "angelic" smile. She was very compassionate and understanding, listening with rapt attention as I responded to her questions. She assured me she would do everything she could to see that I got all the help that was available.

In the end, because of our very limited income, I was fortunate. The Pharmaceutical Companies that manufactured the drugs donated them to me through the Cancer Center, and my Medicaid and Medicare coverage paid for the remainder of my expenses.

I have worked with many social workers over the years, for different reasons and in different settings, and none of them were as friendly, caring and as compassionate as Vikki. Compared to the ones in the hospital and especially in the Department of Social Services, she was a Godsend. I thought that they could definitely take lessons from Vikki on how to deal with clients.

Barbara and I are very blessed indeed to not only have her as my social worker for the cancer center, but to be able to count her as a close friend. Her gentleness and thoughtfulness, and just "being" there has been an inspiration not only to us, but to those she helps each and every day. Sometimes when we least expected it Barbara would get an email that just said hello, thinking about ya, or a call to see how we were doing. They meant a lot to both of us.

A family friend, Peggy Douglas came over to take Barbara and me to the hospital to have the PEG tube inserted. It was a simple in and out surgical procedure. I was not looking forward to going back into the operating room, no matter how briefly. I reported to the Digestive Health Clinic, and had to fill out pages of forms before they called me in. The entire procedure, including the time I spent in recovery, was about 4 hours. I was nauseated and very light-headed when I woke up, and Barbara and Peggy were standing beside my bed. All I knew was I was sick of waking up on those damn hard gurney's, nauseated and feeling worse than when I went in. I was ready to get my clothes on and get out of there right that minute. Unfortunately, they still hadn't taken out the needles from where they had been giving me IV fluids, and I hadn't received my discharge instructions and any prescriptions that they would be giving me.

One of the Nurse Practitioner's in the clinic came in to demonstrate how to clean the site and dress it. She also showed us how to do the tube feeding and flush it after each use. She gave me several cans of the nutritional supplement, and a prescription to pick up several cases at the Hospital Pharmacy. She also gave me a prescription for pain medicine which meant another stop at CVS Pharmacy. They were getting to know me quite well lately.

Finally, home again! Sitting in the car while Peggy went into the pharmacy to fill my medications hadn't helped much. Then the ride had made feel worse than when I was lying down. I was very nauseated and starting to hurt bad since the medication I had gotten at the clinic had, for the most part, worn off. I couldn't wait to sink into the plush cushions of my recliner and kick up the footrest. My stomach was protesting the fact that it hadn't had any food since the night before and I was wondering what I should eat. Anything that would take away that rumbling, nauseated feeling for a while would be welcome.

I knew I definitely wasn't in the mood to fool around with trying to use the tube. I managed to eat some fruits and vegetables and hot soup before sleeping for a good part of the afternoon. I was so used to sleeping on my sides; it took time to learn to sleep on my back. Barbara teased me about cutting enough logs to be stocked on wood for the winter, because I snored so loud.

THE TRIALS OF TREATMENT

The radiation treatments and Chemotherapy began at almost the same time, scheduled to run concurrently for the maximum benefit of reducing the size and growth of the tumor, and I wasn't looking forward to double treatments. I wondered if they would cause even worse side effects or complications with them being so close together. It didn't really matter, because I had no choice if I wanted to beat the cancer and get well. I took a deep breath, and just prayed for the best.

Oh, God! I thought I would hyperventilate the first time the assistant put that mask over my face when I was lying on that cold, gray metal table. When Dr. Reid had first measured me for the mask, it really hadn't seemed like it would be that bad. But then when he proceeded to clamp it down on both sides! It was to prevent me from moving while the radiation was being administered. Talk about nearly freaking out! I felt like an old boar hog trussed up and ready for slaughter. That was as close as I came to experiencing a true panic attack. The mask prevented me from seeing much except what was right in front of me— the machine. The nose piece didn't allow for comfortable breathing, and the mouth piece made it hard for me to talk. But to be clamped down and not being able to move! My heart was beating so fast it actually felt as if it would beat out of my chest.

I didn't realize how close to being claustrophobic I was until that very second, when—with the machine delivering that radioactive burst to zap the tumor—I was held completely motionless on a cold and impersonal slab of steel. I was breathing in short shallow breaths, not taking a deep one until the machine was turned off, and the mask unclamped and removed from my head— AHH, fresh air! It never smelled so, well— ok, even if it was still in the hospital and had the faint hint of medicine. It was free, and I could feel it entering my nostrils, now that they weren't confined and being pinched by the white hard plastic of the mask. I didn't waste any time getting out of there that day. Just to be in the truck and out on the road was a relief after the first day of radiation preparation.

My healthcare team tried to get me an expedited appointment with the Dental Clinic at the University, before the radiation and chemotherapy began. They wanted to be sure that my teeth were clean and that there were no problems with cavities or fillings being loose. But they were booked solid, and I couldn't get an appointment until after I'd received several treatments. Sometimes I would have an early morning radiation treatment, and then would have to go over to Jefferson Park Avenue to see the dentist after lunch, which made for a long day for me.

I eventually had to make many trips back and forth to have fillings that were loose repaired, and I had several cavities that needed to be filled. It had been a long time since I had sat in a dentist chair, which was not exactly my favorite place in the world to be. I wondered if they knew just how painful those long needles were to the sensitive skin in the roof of your mouth and along the gum lines. Or if they ever even thought about it as they pushed and pushed for the Novocain to go in. I also had to have several teeth that were actually pushing against the ones in the front, removed. Yuck! More Novocain and swelled gums and lips for a while until it wore off—what else was I going to have to deal with?

The last step to getting a clean bill of dental health, at least for the time being, was to have a couple of fluoride treatments applied. It would put a protective coating on my remaining teeth so hopefully the radiation wouldn't cause further, more extensive damage. Dr. Grimm also prescribed fluoride trays that had to be put on my teeth every night for 15 minutes each. They were messy and didn't exactly taste the best in the world, but I did them anyway.

As the chemotherapy and radiation treatments continued I began to experience side effects rather more quickly than my healthcare team or I had anticipated. First, I began feeling tired early in the day. I would get out of bed and take a shower before getting dressed. Then Barbara and I would sit in the kitchen catching up on news and having coffee before breakfast. I would eat and then sometimes have to go back and sleep for an hour or so before I felt like doing anything else.

Food was not something I looked forward to with gusto anymore. My stomach was very queasy these days or my appetite just wasn't there, and when I did eat, literally I had to force myself. Everything, even the most delicious meats and vegetables had lost their appeal, tasting more like I had a mouth full of heavy metal, or as if I were chomping down on bland cardboard.

The foods I had really enjoyed and looked forward to eating now made me nauseated to smell them. Foods I hadn't thought of in years held more appeal. To remember what they tasted like I had to close my eyes and visualize it to fully appreciate them. I had no idea that my taste buds would be so affected by the treatments and was disappointed that I couldn't enjoy food anymore.

After a couple of weeks, I started to develop open sores in my mouth, especially in the roof area. I figured—what the hell might as well see how this PEG tube will work. Unfortunately, it didn't go very well. We followed the instructions we were given, and even called the clinic to be sure we were doing it right. It still back-flowed up the tube and caused a big mess.

It would flow back up the tube, shooting out and running all over me and whatever clothes I had on, forcing me to have to wash and change, which drained whatever energy I'd worked up.

I experienced extreme nausea and acidic reflux, with sour water coming up into my throat, and I went through a lot of antacids tablets because of it. After fighting the tube for two or three days always with the same results, I finally told Barbara to forget it, that I was tired of dealing with it.

I decided instead to use Carnation Instant Breakfast, juices, applesauce, fruits and vegetables, and large amounts of mashed potatoes and gravy. Well, it wasn't the food I was used to eating, and it certainly wasn't a "feast" by any stretch of the imagination—but at least I was retaining some nutrients and calories. Barbara would make sure that I ate frequently, sometimes having to push me to eat because I wanted to be stubborn and wait, instead of listening to what my doctors and nutritionist had recommended. Thank goodness she could be stubborn too, or my weight might have dropped off even more than it did. No one seemed to understand that I was frustrated and missed all of the foods I had enjoyed and taken for granted before all of this started. The ones I was forced to eat now weren't what I was used to or even that I particularly liked.

All of the doctors who were on my healthcare team agreed that they didn't want me to risk operating a car while receiving the chemotherapy and radiation, because they had no idea how my body would react to the combination of drugs. They were afraid that if I were driving and had an adverse reaction, I could injure myself or someone else, or even worse if it was during rush hour.

They strongly suggested I have someone drive me to treatments and wait for me everyday. I totally agreed with them, because by this time I was feeling pretty lousy every day and didn't have very much energy. But I did have a big problem. Who could I find that would be willing to take me in to treatment every day of the week and sit there to drive me back home? Sometimes the IV treatments were all day, and other times, I had both radiation and the chemo back-to-back.

Barbara was on Social Security Disability due to Chronic Asthma, and had to go on permanent medical leave in 1989. She spent more time in the hospital than at her job as a telemarketer with a local company. Her Primary Care Physician at the time—Dr. Jeffrey Ligon placed her on permanent medical leave, and told her to apply for Social Security Disability. At that time she had no idea that it would be a three year struggle to be approved. She finally received her disability in 1992.

She had been involved in a vehicle accident in 1999 which totaled the car she was driving and injured her back. The Chiropractor to whom she was referred to sent her to have imaging done on her back, and was the one who discovered that Barbara was suffering from Spinal Bifida. It wasn't until several years later that the condition was properly diagnosed as Degenerative Bone Disease of the spine. Some days, the pain could be so severe she could barely get out of bed, and she found it difficult to move around the house. The pain in her hip made it difficult to do even small tasks when it flared up.

Driving my old truck and having to sit and wait all day in those chairs in the waiting room would have caused her excruciating pain. I know if push had come to shove and I absolutely couldn't drive, and couldn't find anybody else to help she would have done it regardless of how hard it would have been on her. It really upset her that I needed her help and she couldn't be there for me.

She had always hated relying on disability and not being able to do the things that she enjoyed. As time went on and her symptoms worsened, there were times when she became very depressed and would cry from sheer frustration. She had always enjoyed working and hated being cooped up in the house. That was one of the reasons that she loved it when we lived in Charlottesville, until the end of 1998, when we had moved to Greene County to live with her mother. Her mother, after years of being treated for chronic asthma, had been diagnosed with terminal Emphysema and could no longer live alone. When we lived in town, she was active with the church and kept busy with that, and then there was the recycling center, where she would find lots of books that she enjoyed reading. We were both still very active with the church, but I knew she still missed living in town, where access to everything was easier.

Determined I wouldn't have to drive myself because the doctors were against the idea, she telephoned the local Department of Social Services in Orange, VA on March 18th. Barbara wanted to ask them for help with transportation to and from my treatments. Vikki Bravo, my social worker at the cancer center had helped me file applications for Social Security Disability, Supplemental Security Income and

Medicaid so I thought I had all of my ducks lined up, and would get the help I needed. Evidently, even though I had done what was required, I was wrong.

Barbara was put on hold for several minutes which frustrated her. Finally she was transferred to one of the senior eligibility workers for the department. Barbara explained that I was a cancer patient going through chemotherapy and radiation treatments at the University, and that the doctors in charge of my treatments didn't want me to drive because of the side effects that were possible. She also said that we had already filed the applications for Medicaid and Medicare but hadn't received a decision. The worker told her they couldn't help provide transportation for me. When she questioned the woman why, she said it was because my application for Medicaid had not been approved, was not on file, and I didn't have my card yet.

Well! Whose fault was that? It appeared that the Department of Social Services was the one who had dropped the ball. I had carried it on my end, and then they fumbled. What made Barbara and I mad, was that instead of showing compassion for our predicament, the case worker rudely said we would have to find another means of transportation and hung up.

I was shocked and ticked off that she took such an attitude with Barbara when she had been trying to help me. So evidently that meant that they could take the full 45 days to work the case up and we would still have to wait for the card to be generated through the computer system in Richmond and mailed out before they would help me. I was left with no choice; be it right or wrong, physically able or not, I had to drive to the damn treatments every day. Sometimes, I was so weak and nauseated after a treatment, I could barely hold my head up. I would sit and wait for a while before I dared get in the car to drive home. But none of what I had to deal with mattered to them, evidently. My doctors weren't too happy with it when I told them what had happened either.

I took a total of 6 weeks of the oral and IV infusion chemotherapy (and thankfully only threw up three or four times) and had only minimal hair loss. It was mostly at the back of my head near my hairline, and on my neck where the radiation was concentrated the most. That was a good thing, because I was already pretty thin on top, and had started losing my hair when I was in my early twenties. I certainly didn't want to lose any more—if I could help it.

Radiation was a total of 35 treatments, although they had to reschedule a few of the treatments because of nausea and vomiting that prevented me from taking them on schedule. Once or twice, after leaving chemotherapy and making my way to radiology, I would be so nauseated that I would go straight to the nearest bathroom where I would spend more than a few minutes throwing up. Because they had to bolt the mask down to the table, they didn't want to risk my throwing up and possibly choking on my vomit.

Because radiation can dry out your skin and sunlight complicates it further, I was told to stay out of direct sunlight as much as possible during this time. I was agitated, moody, depressed, and bored. I was also so weak I could barely put one foot in front of the other. I would try walking outside in the yard during the early morning hours, or sometimes would just take a cup of coffee out to the picnic table that was under the big tree in our yard to get fresh air and get out of the house. I would be weak as a kitten by the time I got back inside.

What bothered me the most was watching everyone else do things I enjoyed doing like cutting the grass or taking the trash to the dumpsters, (although I did find a way to accomplish that little chore). Barbara would throw the bags of trash on the back of the truck. I would drive and she would toss them into the dumpster! (There's always more than one way to skin the cat, as old-timers used to say).

It bothered the hell out of me watching my brother-in-law, Harold on my riding tractor. He drove from Fluvanna County, after working all week, to spend Sunday working too, with no rest. I felt as useless as an old discarded shoe, and I hated feeling like that.

Barbara was doing all of the housework— the cooking, cleaning, laundry and taking care of me, except for the few times that family and friends pitched in to help. Barbara's ex mother-in-law Peggy came over and cleaned for us once, even washing a few of the inside windows and curtains in both the living room and kitchen. Barbara's aunt, Annie Mae came over and thoroughly cleaned for us twice. My sister Darlene would come with Harold when he cut the grass and she wanted to help and liked to stay busy, and cleaned while he worked outside. We really appreciated what they did to help us, more than they ever realized.

The hardest chore for her was changing the bed linens every day. The radiation treatments had given my skin a burned smell, and along with body oils and sweat, the sheets had a medicinal, hospital smell, plus they had to be changed for sanitary reasons—to prevent rashes or infections. Before the diagnosis, we always shared working on cleaning together, and she would help change the bed, and put the sheets on while I lifted the mattress, which being a queen size was quite awkward and heavy.

With the PEG tube back-filling each time we tried to use it, it made me very nauseated on my stomach and caused gas constantly. It frustrated the hell out of me, because I hadn't wanted to have it inserted in the first place. Dr. Thomas had refused to give me the chemotherapy if I didn't have it done. Now look at me, I thought disgustedly, as I glanced down at the tube sticking out from my stomach, hanging there uselessly. It had put me through another surgery, cost the state more money and for what, to just hang there, irritating me whenever I wore a t-shirt, forcing me to sleep on my sides and back, always having to watch every movement I made, so I wouldn't pull it out or damage it.

We had two full cases of the liquid nutrition sitting on a storage shelf gathering dust that could have been used for a patient who needed it. What a waste! Barbara finally got tired of seeing it sitting there and having to move them to clean. She called the Orange County food pantry and they sent one of their volunteers to come out and pick it up. They really appreciated our thinking of them, because according to the volunteer sometimes they had clients come in who needed that type of assistance.

I quickly became tired of being limited to eating applesauce, fruit and mashed potatoes and gravy, and I was craving real food in any shape or form by now. I had never liked the taste of yogurt, and tried to eat it but—call me a wimp if you want to—to me; it was for women who always watched each and every calorie they pushed past their lips. I needed REAL FOOD, or as close to it as I could get at the moment.

But what would it be? What could I eat that was high in calories, tasted halfway decent and yet be something that I could easily swallow and wash down with lots of liquid? Barbara had some great recipes that she had collected from magazines and products and some that had belonged to her grandmother, and I enjoyed a few but we needed a way to fix more of a variety.

Barbara asked a good friend of hers at church, June Dudley, if she could borrow her electric food chopper, which had a much bigger cup capacity than the small one I had bought for her at Wal-Mart. Sandy donated a new blender someone had given her as a wedding present and she had no plans to use.

One of Barbara's favorite hobbies was collecting recipes and cooking, and she began experimenting with foods, and began to cook bacon, eggs, sausage—anything that she cooked for herself, and would put them into the chopper, grinding them up and putting them on my plate or in a bowl. The smell of real food cooking did whet my appetite again, and I would sit at the kitchen table and enjoy the aromas as she cooked.

The first time she fixed the scrambled eggs and bacon, I thought it was the nastiest thing I had ever seen in my life, but Oh! Did it ever taste like this side of Heaven after eating applesauce and mashed potatoes for so long? It sure didn't take me long to clean the bowl and I actually managed a second helping, washing it all down with coffee and orange juice. One of my favorites was when she would fix me pancakes, and even sausage gravy with biscuits.

The blender didn't get neglected either; Barbara combined Ensure, ice cream, canned fruits (sometimes drained and sometimes not), and ice to make thick creamy milkshakes I could sip through a straw. I didn't like the taste of the Ensure, but over time I became good at ignoring the taste. I knew it was just another obstacle to climb over, and the benefits far outweighed any inconvenience like taste. It had all of the nutrients my body was lacking and the Ensure plus had extra calories too. Fixing the shakes the way she did added even more.

As much as I tried to stay ahead of the weight loss, it happened anyway. I dropped forty-two pounds that my already slender frame could not afford to lose. My doctors, wife and family were really concerned but I was powerless to stop this. We were frustrated because she was preparing high calorie meals and I was drinking anywhere from 4 to 5 of the Ensures a day. So why wasn't I gaining weight? Nobody seemed to have an answer.

In early July, I finally completed the last of both the radiation and Chemotherapies, breathing a huge sigh of relief to have it over with. When I went to Dr. Reibel and Dr. Read for my scheduled appointments, they agreed that the next course of treatment would be to surgically remove the tumor and any damaged tissue surrounding it. They wanted me to rest my body for a while first, and regain strength and stamina, so the surgery wasn't scheduled until mid August

Dealing with Denial

Barbara and I were totally dependent on her Social Security Disability checks each month to pay all of our bills and buy groceries. We were falling farther and farther behind in everything: the electric bill, telephone and cable. We often had to make trips to Madison County to the Skyline Community Action Program for help in paying a cut-off notice on the electric bill. There was a few times that one of the area churches would pay for it for us.

We were still waiting for the Social Security Administration to make a decision on my claim for disability. I had filed for it when I was first diagnosed with cancer in January. I just wondered how long they would take to make their decision; we couldn't keep going on like this indefinitely, because we were running out of places to find help.

We were both worried and stressed out, not knowing which way to turn to come up with a solution. I couldn't expect anyone in my family to help us. My mother was retired and on Social Security, and barely able to make ends meet. The rest of the family, well—they had their own problems I didn't want to know anything about. I had enough of my own to last me a lifetime. My plate was definitely full and threatening to run over.

I called the Department of Social Services in Orange again, although it was the last thing that I wanted to do. I hadn't been able to rely on them for help with anything else I needed, at least not this time.

They had been a big help to me in the past, especially when I had broken my wrist and was out of work while it healed. I had received Food Stamps from the Fluvanna Department of Social Services, which I had really needed at the time. I asked Orange County to mail me an application for Food Stamps and the General Relief Program.

I felt like I had fallen into a time warp and had no way out. I had always worked and made my own way, and it made me feel low, like I had hit rock bottom and had no foothold to crawl out of this bottomless pit. I hated to ask for help from "welfare".

One of the stipulations in the General Relief Application was I had to sign a paper saying I would repay any amount I received from them, when and if my application for Disability was approved. It would be subtracted from any back pay amount I would receive. Damn, the suckers had you coming and going, I though as I signed the paper. Oh, sure—we'll help you, but you'll pay out of the nose for it later! What a joke! A person was damned if they did and damned if they didn't.

We eventually received (what a whopping amount!), $133 in General Relief and $177 in Food Stamps to help us. I know, you're probably thinking I was being greedy, but I wasn't. I just didn't see how $133 a month was going to help us stay ahead of the grim reaper. We were barely making it as it was. There was no way we could pay the bills and buy food and have gas too.

If it hadn't been for friends of ours who took food out of their own cabinets and freezers to help us we wouldn't have had enough to eat during that first winter. And the Commonwealth of Virginia didn't offer any help to those who were struggling due to chronic or debilitating illness beyond their control.

I didn't understand the system, which seemed so full of flaws; it was like a water bucket with holes in the bottom. When you applied for Food Stamps, you were required to also file for Social Security Disability and Supplemental Security Income. Ok, that I could understand no problem.

What I didn't understand, was that once your disability was approved, Social Services dropped all of the assistance they were giving like it was a hot potato. Both of these agencies were originally designed to help the poor people of this country. Yet it seemed more like they worked against each other, not to mention they were definitely working against the people it was supposed to help. It was totally mind boggling to try and figure out. Well, hopefully Social Security wouldn't drag their heels much longer, and we would be alright.

When I went to the mailbox a couple of weeks later, I had finally gotten an official letter from Social Security and went back to the trailer, anxious to tell Barbara about it so we could celebrate the good news. She was sitting in the living room folding a load of laundry when I went in, and she stopped to sort through some of the other mail. I anxiously opened it to find out how much income I would be getting, Barbara watching me—both of us almost giddy with relief that help was on the way. I pulled the letter from the envelope, my eyes scanning the paper quickly, and I did a double take. Surely I had read it too fast and missed something, I thought.

NO, no—this can't be happening I thought in amazement, my eyes blinking rapidly as I read it again, the breath I was exhaling lodging in my throat. They turned down my application for disability! How the hell could they do that? Didn't they realize I had cancer—a debilitating disease that left me totally unable to work? My doctors had verified all of the medical requirements, sending in form after form that they had requested. What the hell are they thinking? Without a word, I held the letter out to Barbara, leaning back and closing my eyes, trying to shut out the feelings of despair that were quickly washing over me.

The reason that they gave for the denial was my education: I was a high school graduate! So, big deal! According to them, I was qualified to work in some type of office setting which wouldn't require a lot of physical endurance and stamina. Physical Endurance and stamina!! What the hell did they know?

What I couldn't believe or understand was exactly when did they expect me to work? I was going to treatments on a daily basis and was so weak it was an effort to hold my head up some days. The nausea threatened to be overwhelming at times, and I was suffering from dry mouth so bad it felt like I had a mouth full of sand. The radiation had "cooked" my salivary glands, leaving them useless. When I wasn't going to radiation or chemotherapy, I had a full schedule of appointments with all of the doctors who were a part of my healthcare team. I had sat around waiting for help from them for nothing! They weren't going to do anything.

Perplexed by my reaction after reading the letter, Barbara reached over and took the papers from my fingers, which felt numb and lifeless as the papers dangled there. As she read the words, her mouth fell open in shock, as tears misted her eyes. "Oh, my God," she exclaimed. She looked over at me, and in a trembling voice, managed to say "Well, we'll just get a lawyer, and appeal it."

With the shock finally wearing off a bit, I felt anger replacing it, and shouted: "What good is that going to do? We might as well forget about it!" I walked out onto the front porch, staring off into space, thinking about what to do now.

As I stood there on the porch staring out into space, I wondered just what the hell we were going to do. There was no way I could even think about going to work, and there wasn't anybody we could ask for help. Dejectedly, feeling as if the weight of the world was on my shoulders, I walked back inside.

Barbara was sitting in the kitchen at the table, and was holding the telephone to her ear, evidently waiting for someone to answer, or she had been put on hold. I couldn't keep from smiling because that was her pet peeve—to be left dangling and having to wait. I poured a glass of Ensure, and grabbing a couple of cookies from the canister, sat down at the table to eat my little pick-me up snack.

Finally, she began speaking, and it took only a couple of sentences before I realized she had called an attorney's office. She was talking to a paralegal and reading the paper to them from Social Security. She listened briefly, and then gave them our phone number, my date of birth, social security number and the phone numbers for Dr. Reibel and Dr. Read. She thanked them and hung up.

She told me she had been talking to the paralegal who worked for Cooper Geraty, the Attorney in Charlottesville she had used to file her appeal for Social Security when it had been denied in 1992. Her lungs had collapsed, reason unknown—although the doctors assumed it was from Chronic Asthma. She had been on full life support twice, first in 1985 for 14 days and again in 1989 for 17 days. They still denied her claim.

It had taken from 1989 until 1992, a court appearance in front of the Administrative Law Judge, two Federal Court appeals, and the intervention of Congressman Virgil H. Goode, Jr. before she actually received her money.

She said they were going to take my case and saw no great difficulty in having the decision overturned. They would be back in touch with us. Yeah, right I thought, we'll see. I just smiled and left it at that because she seemed so damned optimistic about it. I didn't have the heart to bring her back down. But, true to his word, in less than 3 weeks, we received a letter from Mr. Geraty saying my claim had been reviewed and approved! I was totally surprised that he had managed to win the approval in such a short amount of time.

Shortly after that, we got the award letter and learned I would be receiving $909 a month. The money, minus what we owed Social Services and Mr. Geraty, was going to be deposited into our checking account. Of course, you can't expect in this day and time to get good news, without something bad following right on it's heels.

When I received my disability payments, there was a down side to it. In order for us to fall into the guidelines established by Social Security on monthly income, they took Barbara's Supplemental Security Income—$104 away. It wasn't a whole lot of money, but by receiving that check it entitled her to Medicaid, a state run insurance fund for those who fell below the poverty guidelines.

She was forced to give up her Medicaid coverage just so I could receive my disability. She kept telling me that she didn't mind giving it up if it meant I had my checks coming in each month, but it worried me. It was as if it were their way to punish me for applying for and being eligible for benefits. She had been receiving it for so long, and now she lost it so that I would have an income coming in. Life was so unfair at times.

GENEROSITY OF STRANGERS

Once we got the Social Security Disability claim straightened out, we should have been able to relax a little because we had income to pay bills. Well, we did and we didn't. My disability, combined with Barbara's smaller check (since they had taken the Supplemental Security Income away), didn't begin to meet all of our monthly expenses, buy groceries and allow money for gas to get to and from doctor appointments and treatments. The United Way in Charlottesville suggested she call the toll-free number for the American Cancer Society to see if they could offer any assistance. Well, it certainly couldn't hurt, and they might have a program, or would know about something in our area that we could apply for.

Barbara called the American Cancer Society who provided us with three gas cards (similar to credit cards) to help pay for gas It wasn't anywhere near enough and they had a funny way of sending them. They gave us a total of three cards for $50 each. It sounded like a lot, but it was over a period of time. They only sent one at a time and each card was supposed to last for two weeks. Two weeks? I was driving 34 miles a day, 5 days a week. It wasn't nearly enough, and rarely lasted one week. Thank God Vikki was able to write vouchers through the cancer center to the Exxon station on Emmett Street. If not, I wouldn't have had gas go back and forth for the chemotherapy and radiation treatments.

We began to explore other ways to produce extra income, but found nothing suitable because we both had so many physical limitations. Even if we had found something worthwhile, there was no way to do it. I was still on driving restriction and it took all of Barbara's time and energy to take care of me and the housework.

Shortly after Barbara's first husband passed away in 1998, she had been forced to move from the townhouse they shared into a smaller apartment since she was living alone. It was so she would meet the eligibility guidelines of the Section 8 Government Housing Program and the Voucher she was using.

She had begun attending services at a small church that was down-home and had an outreach motorcycle ministry, Living Stones Christian Chapel. It was a "family" oriented church—the pastor and congregation never met a stranger.

They always made everyone feel welcome with a friendly smile and a welcoming hug when they entered the doors, and unlike some churches where you have a dress code to follow, this one was come as you are—and most of the congregation wore blue jeans, vests and boots or tennis shoes. At the time Tommy was still the Pastor and he didn't "preach" at you, but taught you what was in the Bible. Barbara used to tell me that he had a way with whatever he was teaching that day, you always felt as if he were talking right to you. Sandy would also adopt that same style once she took over the ministry.

Barbara quickly became involved with many of their outreach ministry projects, including collecting money and toys for Toy Lift. It was a local charity event held each year to collect toys and gifts for the underprivileged children in the area at Christmas time. One of the ways the church collected money for the event was "donation" jars—at the church and at different businesses around the area.

My mother, who was also looking for a way to help us, suggested we try using the donation jars, asking businesses in the area to help since I was a cancer patient. Hmmm, well it's not what I want to do, I thought, but it just might work. We could give it a shot, couldn't we?

Barbara and I went to visit Peggy, who was living in a mobile home she and second husband, Bill, were renting to buy in Scottsville, VA, a rural part of Albemarle County. She had custody of her son Randy's three children, Michael, Ginnie and R.J.—two of them teenagers, because Randy and his wife Ronda had divorced.

Peggy's husband Bill was a diabetic and a few years her senior. They had married in July of 1989 shortly before Barbara and Peggy's son Ricky married the following month. They were living on a fixed income, between his Social Security and a check he received from the Veterans Administration, because he was a Navy Veteran.

Like ourselves, they looked for ways to supplement their monthly income. When she wasn't cleaning houses, she would hold small yard sales at home with things people gave her that they no longer wanted or were throwing out. We figured if anyone would have jars we could use for our project, it would be her.

Good luck finally smiled down on us when we told her what we were looking for. She had boxes of quart mayonnaise jars that someone had given her to sell in one of her sales that were perfect for what we wanted to do. We sorted through them and gathered a dozen of them and took them inside. She washed and dried them for us while we visited and caught up on how things were going with my treatments and other news.

After the jars had time to dry on the inside, we screwed the lids on tight, (we didn't want to glue them on so we had a way to empty the money), and using a large butcher knife, we cut a wide slot in the lid so folded bills or large coins would slide easily through.

Using a sheet of plain typing paper, scotch tape and a permanent marker, Barbara made a sign: "Dwayne Moore Cancer Fund Any Donation would be appreciated to help a cancer patient pay utility and medical expenses", and attached it to the front of the jar.

Well, now we had the idea and the material, but where were we going to display the jars? On the drive back home, Barbara wrote down every little store and market we passed on a sheet of paper. We were like new-born babes in the woods, not really knowing how to make the idea a reality and we needed to think it through to come up with a plan of action.

We gathered up the local telephone directory, snack foods and drinks and settled down at the kitchen table to get started. The first thing we did was hold hands and say a prayer, for God to guide us in this decision and to reach down and touch the hearts of the people we would ask for help. We began looking for telephone numbers of stores, markets and other possible avenues in our community.

Barboursville is not a large community. It's small in size and population, with a few area attractions to draw in outsiders: a couple of wineries, a resort that had recently received national exposure, but other than that, just a small town in rural Virginia—whose main livelihood was agriculture. We didn't have a lot of options available.

Barbara began calling some of the area businesses and a few were abrupt and uncooperative. I understood that since they didn't know me or my circumstances. We kept calling straight from the telephone book and we finally found two businesses, both with excellent locations who generously donated counter space.

After placing jars at both locations we set out to find more who might be willing to help and we were eventually able to branch out into a larger area. Businesses from Orange to Fluvanna and into Albemarle and Greene Counties became involved in our project. There were three places that were instrumental in helping us that need to be recognized.

The first place was a small convenience store, Mary Lou's (the name has since been changed), and was about five miles from our house. They had a lot going for them: it was on a major highway and in addition to its staples of food and drinks; it also sold gasoline and kerosene, which kept business brisk. There was an in-store deli, where a lot of workers (from the highway department, hunters, and farmers) would stop in for a hot sandwich on cold, blustery mornings, or just a steaming freshly brewed cup of coffee.

We were surprised at how well the donation jar was received, and amazed at the amount people donated each week, sometimes well over a hundred dollars (in bills and lots and lots of change). Barbara and I made a lot of trips to the bank to get wrappers or to cash in change, sometimes just doing a deposit to pay a bill by check.

The second place was in Gordonsville at a local convenience store. At first, I was skeptical about a donation jar there. The manager didn't sound very enthusiastic when Barbara had talked to her on the telephone, but first impressions can be deceiving sometimes. When we went to the store and met her in person, I knew I had been wrong in my opinion of her. Brenda was a brunette of medium build, with warm, brown eyes, very energetic and outgoing.

She asked several questions while we were talking: why I wanted to put donation jars out; if I was receiving any kind of benefits; what I was doing for insurance; and what my prognosis was. She told us about losing her father over a year before to lung cancer, and that it was why she was willing to help. She did suggest we have only one day a week to come in to check and empty the donation jar, and if it needed to be emptied more then she would call us. She preferred that we wait until she was in the store so that her cashiers wouldn't have to work with the jar, and could concentrate on their duties.

For the length of time that we left the jar there, the location helped us the most, often collecting well over $200 a week, and a couple of times we got a call from Brenda to empty it before our scheduled pick up day, and we'd empty it again by the end of the week

My favorite place for a jar has always had a special part of my heart. It is where I spent many days as a child growing up. In a small rural part of Fluvanna County, it was a little corner "market", C.F. Kidd's Store.

It had been owned and operated for years by the same family, and had only recently been sold to a prominent family in the area. The Tapscott's owned a lot of land and real estate in the county, including the logging Company my brother Steve works for.

I remember as a teenager growing up, I bought soda pop and other treats from the store. My maternal grandparents lived next door in a modest two-story frame house.

When the new owners took possession, they left the old family's name on it, and remodeled the inside to also include a deli. It was a welcome addition that was well received in the community. They recently began selling gasoline again that hadn't been available for years. Even though the amount of money we collected in that jar was small in comparison to the others, it still meant a lot to me.

If it had not been for my mother thinking of the suggestion, our donation jar project may never have materialized nor provided much needed assistance. I often felt embarrassed going into the businesses to empty the jars. I felt as if every eye in the place were watching me, and thinking I was doing it because I didn't want to work. Or maybe they thought it was some other "underhanded" reason. It just made me angry to do it. Then I would think of how many people had kind hearts, donating because they seemed to understand how cancer could affect a person's life, and I was grateful for their generosity.

In April, our Church, Living Stones Chapel was preparing to hold a yard sale (which they did periodically throughout the year in good weather) to raise money for repairs and church supplies. People from all over the area would use the sale as an excuse to clean out closets, dressers, garages and attics, and sometimes the basement entrance to the church would be piled so high from stuff people had dropped off, that it would have to be moved down to the shed before you could unlock the door.

The weather had been very uncooperative all spring, and the yard at the Church often had "rivers" of water standing in it. It was hardly a day that went by we didn't have severe thunderstorms. It prevented any vehicle from driving to the shed at the back of the church property.

Finally, a week of sunshine and warm breezes helped soak up the water and dry the grass so that June called Barbara and said she and Sandy were going to be cleaning out the building the next day. Barbara offered to help sort and clean the items for the sale and we made arrangements to meet them there mid morning.

Did we ever receive a shock when we arrived at the church? They already had enough volunteers to clean out the building, and since it didn't appear that they had anything at the moment they needed our help with, Barbara and I walked inside to talk to Sandy and June, who were in the office.

When we walked in, June said that she and Sandy had talked about it and decided they weren't going to include the clothing and some of the other stuff that had been donated in their sale and that they wanted us to have it. Barbara and I thought it would be enough clothing that maybe she would find a few things for us and we could share it with a few friends. Sometimes it just doesn't pay to jump to conclusions.

By the time they had completely gotten everything out of the building and separated, I had hauled two full loads of stuff to our house, and it was beginning to look like I was going to almost have a full third load. There were mountains of black trash bags, white smaller bags, boxes and even totes full of stuff. I didn't have time to find a place to pack it away, and had just tossed it all onto the front deck at the house.

When we were getting ready to pull out a short time later, Sandy came over to the truck and said we were more than welcome to "piggy-back" a yard sale with them that coming weekend. Was Sandy referring to this weekend coming up, the one that was two days away? Uh, ho, that meant a lot of stuff to get through and organize in just two days! We told her that we would like to do it, and that we would put something together for at least a small one. Were we up to it? Time would tell.

When we got home, Barbara was shocked at the amount of stuff that I had piled onto the front deck, and just stood there shaking her head in total disbelief. I still hadn't unloaded what they tossed on the truck before we left, which I wasn't sure would fit on top of the other stuff.

We went into the house to change into old clothes and to get something cold to drink before we went out to the front deck to get started on the sorting process.

Barbara and I both worked on that mountain of clothes outside on the deck until dark, and then we moved some of it inside to the living room. We had clothes and other items strewn all over the floor and on every piece of furniture in the room as we rushed to get enough to put into that sale. We worked late into the night and then tackled it after breakfast the next morning. Somehow we managed to get it all sorted out and boxed by the end of the week.

By the grace of God we put that sale together with a lot of hard work, and Sandy loaned us tables from the Fellowship Hall downstairs. We also used ply board that she had available, laying it over wooden saw benches to make wide tables so that we were able to put out a lot of items. We were amazed by the end of the sale two days later that we had made over $300.

I knew God had been with us throughout the diagnosis and all of the treatments I had endured and come through, and He gave us the strength to survive each and every pitfall. Our faith and prayers were being answered in ways we'd never imagined and we were truly blessed. It says in the Bible that with God all things are possible. You'd better believe it. Barbara and I were walking, talking living proof. By trusting in Him, He had provided a way for us to meet all of our needs and obligations.

My birthday is July 19, and my zodiac sign is Cancer. I thought that we would be spending just a quiet day at home, the two of us, maybe watching television or just napping and relaxing. I was sure in for a nice surprise by the end of the day.

As my birthday approached, Barbara, without my knowledge talked to all of my family and they made plans for everyone to come up to our house and spend time with me here.

Barbara baked me a cake and my mother went by Food Lion and bought one and had my name put on it. My mother, my sister Darlene and her husband Harold, my sister Linda and her husband Sean, my nephew Brian and his wife Melissa, and, my niece Chrissy all came by, along with my brother Steve. I was really surprised because I didn't know they were going to do this. Barbara had gone out of her way to surprise me and I know she was trying to cheer me up and help me forget about all of the stuff that was going on. The best part of it wasn't just the company. I got some pretty cool gifts too.

I'm a big NASCAR fan and a die-hard Dale Earnhardt fan, and after Dale, Sr. was tragically killed at the 2001 Daytona 500, I started following his son Dale Earnhardt, Jr., who drives the #8 Budweiser Chevrolet. I still collected memorabilia from either driver.

My family surprised me by giving me model car kits you put together with glue and can paint them. They said they knew I would be bored having to sit around the house, so they wanted me to have something to look forward to working on to occupy my time. I loved them and couldn't have gotten anything any better. I'd never really done much with model cars before and was looking forward to it.

My sister Darlene really surprised me, because she had found a model kit of the #8 Budweiser Chevrolet. Hot DOG! I knew which one I was going to be putting together first. And I had the perfect place to display it. Right on top of the television so I could see it while I was relaxing in my recliner.

UNDER THE KNIFE

As the hot and humid days of August began to melt one into the other, Barbara and I were thinking of the upcoming surgery scheduled for August 18. We talked about it, thought about it, and wondered what side effects I would have to deal with once it was over. Would I have to have a tracheotomy? Would removing the cancer damage my vocal chords? Would it affect the sound of my voice in any way? There were so many unanswered questions and things that we didn't know.

I still had to meet for the final time with Dr. Reibel. The only thing we knew was that he would be removing the mass at the back of my throat, and neither one of us had any idea what could be involved in doing that. Hopefully when I went in for the appointment he would be able to answer some of the questions when he explained how the surgery was done.

After being under anesthesia for other procedures, it didn't frighten me being sedated. But I was worried about what they would do and what they would find once they were inside my throat. Although the pathology report had staged it and concluded that it was non-malignant, there was always the distinct possibility that during the tonsillectomy in February they had missed something and it would show up when they went in to remove the mass.

Ten days before the surgery, I went to my appointment, and Dr. Reibel explained the procedure. It was called a lateral neck dissection.

He said it was routine for him and his team, and that they had successfully performed hundreds over the past few years. I was glad to know that, but it didn't calm the nervous anticipation that seemed to be controlling my thoughts and feelings more and more with each passing day.

How would it affect my speech, swallowing, looks, feelings; thousands of questions seemed to fight with each other to get out, and yet—uneducated in what to ask, I didn't utter a word. I did what he told me to do; I went where he told me to go and left the rest to him

I was still unable to drive, so June Dudley, a friend and church member, offered to drive us to the hospital. She works as a van driver for Open Door Christian School in Fluvanna County. I needed to be in the Admissions waiting room at 11:45 a.m. It had never occurred to Barbara or me when we made the arrangements for June to drive us in that day, how Barbara would get back home with no transportation. I knew that she didn't consider it important because she was planning on staying there at the hospital with me overnight. I wasn't sure if the hospital staff would allow that or not, but I was sure that Barbara would find a way to make it possible if she could. Most of the time, when serious surgeries were involved; the hospitality staff would bring a cot to the patient's room for one family member to spend the night.

According to the instructions the nurse had given Barbara the previous day, I could only have small sips of water or coffee without cream or sugar. I was wishing it had been scheduled for earlier in the day, because my stomach was growling something fierce from lack of food. I was so nervous that it was probably a good thing that I wasn't allowed to have anything to eat because it wouldn't have stayed down for very long anyway.

June got to our house around 11 a.m., coming from home after exchanging the van for her personal car. Within a few minutes, we were on our way to Charlottesville. I had taken a shower and washed my hair, although they had told me to be sure not to use any kind of oil or conditioner prior to going into surgery, and I was dressed and ready to go when she knocked at the back door.

There had been construction crews working on Route 29 all week, but I didn't think to suggest she take the back way. We got stuck in a traffic jam, and with the clock ticking, I knew we'd never make it on time. Barbara used June's cell phone and called ahead to let them know we were on our way and would be there as soon as possible.

We got through the traffic jam without incident, but as we were approaching the University area, a car pulled directly into our path without yielding the right of way. It took quick reflexes for June to avoid it, and we got a good laugh. I could have ended up in the Emergency Room from an accident instead of surgery.

June drove up to the main entrance for us to get out, since she wasn't planning to go in with us She had a couple of errands to run before driving the children home from school that afternoon. We hugged, and Barbara promised to keep her updated with any news.

Barbara had packed a small overnight bag for me since I would be staying after the procedure. I have never liked the open backed gowns so my mother had bought me a couple pairs of pajamas, and Barbara packed those and my bedroom slippers and robe, then a few toiletries that I would need. She would leave the clothes I had on at the hospital for me to wear back when they discharged me. As we moved toward the Admissions waiting room, we held hands, trying our best to calm each other down and failing miserably. Looking at us, it would have been hard to tell which one of us was more nervous.

After being tied up in the traffic jam, we were twenty minutes late arriving, and I was called as soon as I gave my name at the receptionist desk. I had a wheelchair for Barbara, since she couldn't walk long distances without either having to rest or move very slowly when her back gave out, which made her legs weak and hard to walk.

Like with the biopsy I had earlier in the year, I undressed and Barbara put my clothing into a hospital bag and helped me into the booties, gown and cap patients were required to wear in surgery. Glancing down at it I joked that it didn't seem to be my color, causing her to smile through watery eyes that threatened to spill tears any second. I had left my watch at home because I couldn't wear jewelry in surgery, and it upset me that I had to remove my wedding band. Barbara took it and put it behind hers, promising to put it back on for me when I got upstairs.

A member of the surgical team came in to introduce himself, and explained briefly how the procedure would be done. He said I should be out of surgery in about an hour and a half. The Recovery Room team would call downstairs when I was awake and alert.

Barbara and I hugged and kissed, and I could tell she was having a hard time not breaking down completely. I stretched my hand out; touching hers yet again when they began wheeling me out of the cubicle toward the operating room. I mouthed "I love you" and gave her thumbs up as the gurney slid through the double doors, closing us off from each other. "Lord," I prayed silently, be with the doctors today for a successful surgery, and please watch over my wife until I'm with her again, Amen".

As the orderlies pushed me through those wide double doors and into the operating room, it sure looked a lot bigger and more menacing to me than it had when I was working here as a house keeper. Then it dawned on me. Back then, whenever I had come in here, it had been walking on my own two feet and not lying stretched out on a bed on wheels. They pushed me over to the operating table, with the large bright lights hanging down from the ceiling over it. I managed to take a calming breath, and scoot from the gurney into the middle of the table, positioning myself where they directed, and having one of the nurses cover me.

Once I had been put under by the Anesthesiologist, the surgeons opened my throat and removed 40 lymph nodes from the left side. They were lying against where the tumor was located; and they didn't want to take chances that even one of the nodes had been compromised. If it had and they didn't remove it there was a possibility that if it were infected with a cancer cell, it could travel and spread (they called it metastasize) to other parts of my body.

To reach the mass, they had to carefully dissect several areas of my throat. They removed the mass by cutting the Sternocleidomastoid Muscle (which controls the movement of my left arm and shoulder, and the ability to turn my neck from one side to the other), and then reconnected the nerves.

They also cleaned the area where the tumor had been lodged, removing as much of the damaged tissue as possible. They were hoping it would save having to go back in to remove it at a later time.

I knew that it was going to be a long and very emotional day for Barbara, as she sat there, waiting to hear from the team of doctors performing surgery. I could only hope she knew I was there with her in spirit. I will let her tell what it was like for her that day.

Barbara's View of the Day of Surgery:

I tried hard all day, from the time we got out of bed that morning, not to let Dwayne see how upset I was. We've been together for so long and have experienced more than our fair share of heartaches and tragedy. We can tell what the other is thinking and feeling without words being spoken. Sometimes it could be very difficult.

I could have drunk a whole pot of coffee that morning without stopping, but I never brewed the first one. It would have gone a long way to helping me wake up and to calm my nerves. I didn't want to be enjoying a cup in front of Dwayne when he couldn't have more than a sip to wet his lips and throat. It wouldn't have been fair to him. This whole mess we were in the middle of seemed unfair anyway and I wasn't going to add to it. I would get me a cup or two later at the hospital while I was waiting for news.

On the drive to the hospital, my knees were shaking as I sat in the front seat of June's car. I couldn't help but worry what would happen once he was on the operating table. What if something went wrong? I tried not to think negative thoughts, but somehow they kept sliding into my thoughts. I was truly thankful for the long line of the traffic jam, because it postponed, at least for a little while, the fact I would have to watch him being wheeled into the operating room.

Not knowing what could happen when he was out of my sight, lying on that cold operating table with the team of doctors cutting into his flesh, searching for the cancer and the damage it had caused, had me very worried. I knew that the doctor had assured Dwayne that it was more like a routine procedure to them because they did a lot of it. But this was different. I hadn't known any of the other people that they had operated on. Dwayne was my husband, my soul mate and my best friend. I would be lost if something were to happen to him. He had been my rock for so long, always there for me when I needed him the most. We tried to be there for each other, and right now I was feeling pretty damn useless. There was nothing I could do to help him through this except to pray and be there to help him when he needed me.

My heart skipped a couple of beats when the nurse came through the door on the opposite side of the waiting room and called his name as soon as he gave it at the receptionist's desk. Closing my eyes and taking a deep breath, I watched him pick up the overnight bag from the floor, and place it on my lap. As our eyes connected he began pushing my wheelchair and walking toward her. Each step was taking us closer and closer to the unknown, and I felt a knot of tension sink into the pit of my stomach.

Evidently the nurse was used to walking and working at a fast pace, because Dwayne had to rush to keep up with her. She led us around to the staff elevators, and as the doors closed, I heard him breathing hard from the exertion. I reached my hand up and placed it over his, giving it a firm squeeze. Tilting my head back I tried to give him a smile which fell flat.

When we got to the second floor, the nurse pushed the wide sensor plate on the wall to open the heavy doors of the Operating Suite, and they opened much quicker than I remembered from when I used to come up and visit him when he was working here as a house keeper. We walked through the doors as they closed rapidly behind us. It sounded like a loud clap of thunder as they clanked shut, sealing us inside. I felt a shiver slide down my spine as we followed the nurse to the cubicle that had been assigned to him.

I got out of the wheelchair in the hallway outside of the curtained cubicle. It was a tiny space, and I didn't want to be falling over the chair as I helped Dwayne get undressed. There was barely enough room for the gurney style bed, and the small steel beside table and a very uncomfortable looking wooden chair. It felt like the hands of the clock went into a whirlwind, with the seconds and minutes flying by, until they came and wheeled him away.

One of the nurses was really sweet and seemed to understand how hard it was for me to deal with. She came over and brought a box of Kleenex and a wet cloth to wash my face. She said she would take me back downstairs to the waiting room after I pulled myself together. I really appreciated her kindness, and I quickly gulped down air to settle my nerves, frantically drying the tears from my eyes. I was beginning to feel claustrophobic.

I didn't want to be inside that suite another minute, and was starting to feel like I couldn't breathe, and she dropped what she was doing to take me back. She talked to me while on the elevator, and I know it was her way of trying to get me to think of other things, and I appreciated her thoughtfulness. I thanked her with as bright a smile as I could muster when she turned to leave.

I know you're probably going to think I'm crazy, considering I have chronic asthma, and Dwayne was upstairs in surgery for throat cancer, and I probably was. The only thing I could think of was to walk outside to the enclosed smoking area and enjoy a couple of cigarettes. The doctors had never really determined what had caused the cancer, although like most doctors do, they contributed it to the fact that he had been a smoker for the past several years and that he enjoyed his beer.

After telling the receptionist I was stepping out for a few minutes, that is exactly what I did. I stopped by the bathroom first to wash my face. I was so nervous, the lighter shook as I held it to the tip of the cigarette, and a woman sitting beside me lit it for me. Smiling at her gratefully, I leaned back on the bench closing my eyes, as I enjoyed that cigarette. For some reason, maybe just being on the outside of those doors, I felt a little calmer than when I had walked out.

I sat there for about half an hour before going into the cafeteria for a cup of coffee. I needed the jolt of caffeine to settle my nerves, and was used to drinking several cups before starting my day. There is a rule about no food or drink being allowed in the waiting room early in the day. There are people who are scheduled for surgery and who couldn't have anything by mouth still there, waiting to be taken upstairs for their procedures.

I fixed my cup of coffee and paid for it, and leaving the cafeteria, had to take my time to walk back to the waiting room. My back was hurting by now, so I stopped at the pay phones to rest. By the time I walked into the waiting room all of the patients had been called upstairs. The only ones in here now were family members and friends. Some were sleeping while others chatted on their cell phones or read magazines and books. How can they be so calm and relaxed I remember thinking to myself? Here I am feeling like I'm about to jump out of my skin and they're as cool as a cucumber.

I was too nervous to do much except fidget as I slowly sipped my coffee. Every time the telephone on the wall rang, I'd nearly jump out of my skin. Finally, I realized that the day was going to be long enough and I needed to find something to occupy my time. The waiting room had a couple of computer stations set up on one side, and I tried to concentrate and play games, but that didn't go over too well, and thankfully you could delete your scores.

Dwayne's family, friends, his stepchildren, all of them called, wanting to know if there was any news. Afraid that the staff working the waiting room would get mad because I had so many calls coming in,

I finally told them I wasn't the only one there waiting for news, and that I would call his mother when I knew anything and she could relay the news. This was also the phone where the doctors and nursing staff from upstairs called so I couldn't keep it tied up. I didn't have a lot of money with me to keep feeding the pay phone out in the lobby either.

During that long day I cried, I talked to myself and I prayed over and over again as I sat there. I would take time out every couple of hours to go outside to stretch my legs and have a cigarette, or buy another cup of coffee before coming back. Around 3:00, his step-daughter, Tina and granddaughter Amber, came up to bring me lunch and to see if there was any news. I was beginning to get worried as the receptionist cleared off the desk, preparing to leave for the day, and there was still no news. I could only hope and pray that something hadn't happened in the operating room and that Dwayne was alright.

Finally, at 5:30 the phone on the wall rang, and Dr. Reibel was on the other end. He apologized for not letting me know what had been happening, quickly assuring me Dwayne came through the surgery with flying colors, and was now in recovery. He went on to explain why it had taken much longer than he had anticipated in surgery.

When they had finally dissected the inside and gotten to the tumor, it had a nerve wrapped around it that had to be carefully moved. They had had no other choice but to sever the Sternocleidomastoid muscle during surgery. I wondered to myself what the Sternocleidomastoid muscle was, and told myself I would ask him when I saw him in person. They had also taken out all of the scar tissue around the site where the tumor was located so that it would reduce the risk of having to go back in at a later time. He said that he and the team were surprised Dwayne hadn't bled more than a teacup full during the surgery, and that he was already awake, alert and asking for ice. When I heard Dr. Reibel say that made it me feel a little better. The fact that Dwayne had come through the surgery without any major complications was such a huge relief to me, and I was anxious to see for myself. Dr. Reibel gave me the unit and room number where he would be transferred to from the Recovery Room.

I gathered up the few things that I had brought with me for the day, cleaning up the tissues and coffee cups from the table and throwing them away. I went to the bathroom and then washed my face and hands before going outside to smoke a cigarette. Dr. Reibel had said that it would be a little while before they brought Dwayne upstairs because they were still waiting for the room to be cleaned by house keeping and for transportation to come for him. It was almost two hours later before transportation brought him to his room. I had been asking the nurse at the nurses' station how much longer she thought it would be when I turned and saw them bringing him down the hallway. He was so pale and white in the face and I could tell he was in pain by the expression he wore. I could see the drains they had left in, and they were already filling with drainage and blood. I waited out in the hallway until they had gotten him situated in bed before walking into the room.

Dwayne looked so small lying in that big hospital bed, surrounded by those white sheets. I couldn't help but cry, tears sliding silently down my cheeks as I said a silent prayer, thanking God for bringing him through the surgery safely. I walked over to the bed, drying my eyes on my hands as I gave him a watery smile, and leaned over to kiss his cheek, which felt warm to the touch.

Dwayne's View:

I could hear the hustle and bustle around me, people talking in low whispers, water being poured into pitchers or glasses long before I could summon the energy to open my eyes. My eye lids felt like there was a paperweight holding them closed, and I had to rest for a while before I made the effort to open them. It took a little more work than I expected to get them open, and my eyelashes felt gritty, wet with matter from having them closed for so long I suppose. As I became more aware of my surroundings, my mouth felt parched and gummy, making it hard to pry my lips apart. It was as if someone had super glued them together while I was asleep. I cautiously opened my eyes, blinking rapidly against the light to bring them into focus.

A nurse was standing beside my bed and was reading the monitor attached to my finger for oxygen and was recording my blood pressure from the automatic cuff that had started inflating when I first became aware of my surroundings. After jotting down the information on my chart she smiled a bright friendly smile and asked me how I was feeling.

For the life of me I couldn't get my mouth open enough to utter one word. I just blinked several times at her, helpless to do anything else. She quickly disappeared momentarily around the curtained cubicle, returning with a wet washcloth. Leaning over, she very gently used it to moisten my parched lips, which felt so good I sighed in relief, closing my eyes as she slid it over each lip.

Once I could open my mouth, I managed to ask if I could have some ice chips, and she said I couldn't have anything until they determined I wasn't going to vomit. She said she could give me a couple of pre-moistened swabs to hydrate the inside of my mouth. I could only nod in agreement as my eyes followed her to where they were stored in a cabinet. Taking them from her, I opened my mouth and slowly rubbed the swab around my tongue, the inside of each cheek and along my gum lines, before placing it on the small table in front of me.

When I finally became aware of the time, I found it hard to believe it was almost six O'clock in the evening. I gasped in shock, never realizing that the entire day had slipped by and my hand immediately moved up to feel my throat, as I glanced at the nurse with wide eyes. She immediately sensed my panic because she hurried to assure me everything was alright, and that the surgery had been successful.

She said they had taken out scar tissue while they were inside to prevent another surgery later on. Taking a deep breath and trying to relax, I asked," what about my wife?" She told me that Dr. Reibel had talked to Barbara and that she would be waiting for me when I got upstairs. After what seemed like an eternity, two people from transportation arrived and took me upstairs to the rehabilitation unit on six East. I looked puzzled, and they explained it was the only bed available at the moment, and my doctor might decide to transfer me when another bed became available.

Barbara, who was looking very tired and worried, was standing at the nurse's station, talking with someone when they wheeled me down the carpeted hallway to the room. Our eyes met and I tried to smile at her, but the pain medication they had been giving me in recovery was beginning to wear off, and I hurt so bad all I could think about was getting through it for the moment. As the orderlies pushed me into the room, I saw her beginning to walk down the hallway toward me. She waited outside of the room until they had transferred me into the bed and left before coming over to my bedside.

The nurse who would be in charge of my care for the rest of that day until the middle of the night came into the room and asked the routine questions to fill in her part of the chart. Barbara had already brought the overnight bag in and stored the stuff in the closet, and since I wasn't going to be needing it, she would keep my wallet with her so I didn't have any valuables that they needed to list, other than my wedding band which Barbara had already placed back on my finger after I asked for it.

With the drains left in place, I had to lie on my back. They wanted me to lie flat; but I finally convinced the nurse who came into the room to adjust the head of the bed a little and to fluff the pillows so my head was at least a little elevated. Barbara wanted to touch and hug me but she was afraid to because of the drains and lines from the IV's that were in the top of my hand. I have always hated when they put them there. As many veins as a person has on their body, they always seemed to make a beeline for the hand. I guess it was because they were easy to slip that damn needle in without much work. But they hurt like hell and made the pump beep if you so much as twitched a finger.

When I asked for ice chips, the nurse said that she wouldn't be able to give me any until she had the chance to call my doctor for permission. She asked a lot of routine questions I didn't want to deal with because I was feeling dehydrated and was in pain. Evidently, according to the nurse, I would have to tough it out for a little while. I wasn't scheduled for another dose for an over an hour.

I knew that Barbara, stubborn as she was, would never admit how tired she was or how much her back was hurting her. She would just tough it out, and stay there in the room with me all night. I loved her for wanting to do that, but I was in so much pain I didn't want her to see how bad it was. I was trying not to make any sound, holding it back because it was an effort to just groan at the moment. She sat in the chair beside the bed, holding my hand.

I told her she should call someone to pick her up and go home. She could get some rest and come back the next day. She tried to argue, but I wouldn't let her. It took all of my energy to assure her that I would be alright. I even managed a smile to convince her. I could tell as she chewed on her bottom lip that she was having a hard time trying to decide what to do. Reluctantly, she finally agreed, and called Tina. She could stay with her stay with her overnight and Tina would bring her back to see me the next day. She had already been here at the hospital too long, and it would do her good to get away for a while. She could always use the phone to call and check on me.

After Barbara left to go downstairs to wait for Tina to pick her up, I closed my eyes and tried to concentrate on getting through the pain until it was time for my next dose of medication. God, why did they space out giving it to you after something major like cutting open your throat, I wondered. I tried to count my breaths just to have something to concentrate on. Finally opening my eyes to glance at the clock on the wall, it was just a few minutes left to go and I pushed the nurse's button to summon help. I kept pushing that damn button over and over for what seemed like an eternity, but was probably no more than an hour, and nobody came in to see what I needed. I was frantic. The pain was unbearable by now, and I did the only thing I could think of. I managed to dial Tina's number.

Barbara answered the phone because Tina was fixing supper and I whispered as loud as I could manage that I needed help. She asked me what was wrong and I told her they still hadn't given me any pain medication and weren't coming in when I signaled for help. I managed to get the phone hung back up.

I was a man, 54 years old and I suppose some people would call me a coward, and I admit I probably was at that point. But I also knew that when she found out how much pain I was in, and that the nurses on the floor were ignoring me, she would come to my rescue and see that I got my medication. After hanging up the phone, I closed my eyes, determined to hang in there until help arrived. Knowing Barbara, she would probably make Tina walk out the door as soon as she got off of the phone.

About 45 minutes later, my room had suddenly transformed into a beehive of activity. My medication had been given to me, fresh water filled the pitcher on the bedside table, along with a cup of ice chips and a spoon, and my sheets, blanket and pillows had been fluffed up. Nurses were walking in and asking if I was comfortable or if there was anything else I needed. I wondered what in the world had happened when Barbara had gotten back to the hospital. What had changed their attitude?

I didn't find out until the next morning what had happened. Once they gave me the medication, I dozed off into a drug-induced sleep.

Barbara had gotten to the hospital after visiting hours, which meant that she technically was supposed to have an overnight pass to be on the floors. She had gone to school with the security guard who was on duty, and he let her slide by without one. When she confronted the nurse at the station she was told that they were on their coffee break at the moment. When she glanced down and saw the light constantly flashing over my door, she asked how long they had been on one.

Evidently the answer didn't sit too well with Barbara, and she asked them to page Dr. Reibel for her. The nurse had an attitude and told her that Dr. Reibel didn't have anything to do with that floor because he wasn't the attending in charge. Barbara nearly exploded and told her he might not have anything to do with the floor, but he sure as hell had something to do with me and that she wanted him paged. When the nurse refused, Barbara jerked up the receiver of the phone and paged him herself.

She waited on the phone while the operator paged him, and when he came on the line, she explained to him why she was calling. She had left for the night and had to come back because I was in excruciating pain and not getting my medication, and that the nurse had an attitude. He said that he would be right up, and she hung up the telephone. Dr. Reibel is very protective of his patients and he came marching down the hallway like one of the guards at Buckingham Palace. He definitely took a very harsh attitude with the nurses and was so loud in doing it, that he actually woke up Dr. Read, who had been asleep in one of the on-call suites on the floor. His attitude must have shaken them up enough for them to forget about drinking coffee, because I didn't do without my medication any more that night.

I woke up early the next morning and Barbara was sitting in the chair at my bedside looking at a magazine. I smiled at her when she stood up after realizing I was awake. I was disoriented and groggy from the morphine and it took me a few minutes to shake the cobwebs out enough to really focus on things around me. I managed to ask her how long she had been there, and wasn't really very surprised when she said she had spent the night. I knew when she had found out they didn't give me my medicine she wouldn't leave for the rest of the night.

Barbara went out to the room to where the ice machine is located and got some fresh water and a cup of ice chips, feeding me a few to wet my lips and mouth, so that it was more comfortable to swallow. The nurse came in and took all of my vital signs, and Barbara got a wet washcloth to clean my face and hands which made me feel a little better.

The pain was noticeable even with the morphine but at least it was bearable. The nurse told us when she came in that they would begin tapering down the amount I was getting through the IV, and start giving it to me in tablet form so I could get used to swallowing it before I was discharged. It took me a few tries to get the first dosage to go down since my throat was sore and very irritated, as well as being dry as a chip.

One of the first questions I asked the nurse when she came back into the room was if they would be bringing me breakfast and what time they served it. I had not had anything to eat since the night before surgery and my stomach was growling so loud I knew anyone standing close could hear it. I didn't know how I would swallow anything but I was definitely going to give it my best shot. The server finally brought it a little after 8:00. I had oatmeal, buttered toast, orange juice and Jell-O. I know most people would have frowned at being given such a breakfast but it looked real good to me and I started with the oatmeal, which I thought would be the easiest. It took me over an hour to finish it but I ate every morsel. I would have loved to have had a cup of coffee, but I was scared it would be too much on my throat. I had the orange juice instead.

Barbara moved the tray over to the air conditioning unit so that the table was cleared except for the water and things I was using. It was hard for me to move my arm, and she lowered the tray. She moved it to the right side of the bed so it would be easier for me to reach things on it.

One of the personal care attendants came in with fresh linens for the bed and said that she was there to help me take a sponge bath. I wasn't too keen on the idea, but agreed to it. While she was helping me with that Barbara stepped out to go down to the cafeteria for a sandwich and a cup of coffee. The doctors had made arrangements for her to get vouchers for meals so she wouldn't have to spend money on food.

After the assistant finished with my bath, she put me into the hospital gown even though I tried to tell her that I had pajamas in the closet. She said that the gowns would be more comfortable with me lying in bed and easier for the nurses when it came to dealing with the IV lines and all. What did she know? I hated those gowns and wanted my pajama's on. She helped me scoot over to sit in the chair so she could change and remake the bed.

As I gingerly laid back on the fresh linens she said that the doctors had put on my chart that they wanted me to get up and walk around some today. What, walk around, I thought, wearing this gown with my back side shining for everybody to see? No way, forget about it! I refused to budge from the bed. She looked exasperated as she walked toward the door, mumbling under her breath that she would tell the nurses.

When Barbara got back from downstairs with her sandwich and coffee, she wanted to know why they hadn't used my pajamas instead of the gown. She said that after she ate she would ask the nurse what she thought. The nurse thought that pajamas would make me feel better, especially if I was out of bed, so she and Barbara worked together to help me into them.

The breakfast, bath, getting out of bed for it to be changed, and then getting my pajamas on had worn me out. I slowly drifted off to sleep for over an hour. Barbara called everyone to let them know how I had done the night before and how I was feeling this morning. When I woke up I felt a little refreshed and was hungry again. The nurse brought me a cup of vanilla ice cream which helped for the time being. As I finished it I wondered what lunch would be.

I had quite a few visitors that day including Tina and Amber, my mother, and my sister Darlene and her husband, Harold. They brought me fruit, ginger ale's, get well balloons, cards and the best thing of all, a creamy chocolate milk shake! Oh, did that ever taste cold, smooth and delicious sliding down! I sat propped up in bed enjoying it while everyone talked around me, and I would answer questions or make short answers since it was still hard to talk a lot at one time. After everyone left, I took a short nap. The milkshake had filled my stomach and the medicine had made me too sleepy to hold my eyes open.

Transportation ordered a wheelchair for Barbara, and holding to the back of it, we made a walk around the floor, but it was slow going. I was weak and unsteady on my feet, having to stop several times to rest. The wheelchair was certainly a good thing for both of us on that trip. A part of me wanted to keep walking around, but I knew I couldn't overdo it the first time I was out of bed. I was really glad to get back to my room and the bed. It wasn't comfortable, and felt more like I was lying on a slab of concrete, but it was still better than trying to stand or walk, and I didn't have the energy to sit up either.

Late Saturday afternoon Dr. Reibel came in to check on how I was doing. After looking at the surgery site, he put on gloves and removed the drains that he had left in as a precaution. He got my chart out of the door, and read over my vitals and food and liquid intake for the day.

Evidently it impressed him because he said that he felt like if I continued improving I could go home the following afternoon.

That was the best news I had heard all day. Thank God! Yes. Home! My own bed, food, and no constant needle pricks, temperature and blood pressure checks—everything that prevented a sick person from sleeping! Sometimes it seemed as if I had just dozed off to sleep when a nurse would wake me up taking my blood pressure or temperature, or they would shake me gently to tell me it was time for my pain medication. After they left the room it would take me a long time to fall back to sleep, only for it to start all over again.

By the time I saw Dr. Reibel, Barbara had already gone home to clean the house. The environment I would be in had to be as germ and dust free as possible over the next few weeks while my body recuperated and my strength returned. My immune system had been severely compromised with the removal of the lymph nodes and it was the best way to guard against my contracting any sort of infection.

Amber, who I admit I spoiled more than I should have whenever I was around her, wanted to do something to help her granddaddy. She spent the night helping clean the kitchen, living room and especially our bedroom. They dusted, vacuumed, changed the sheets, and spread so that it would be ready when I got home the following day.

Barbara and I talked several times over the phone that afternoon and evening. She would ask if I had everything I needed. She really didn't have a way to get back over there but if it had been important, I'm sure she would have found a way. She had proved that the night before. She is very defensive when it comes to me and always has been since we've been together. I can't fault her for being that way because I am the same way where she is concerned.

Discharge and Effects

I was awake quite early on Sunday morning, watching as dawn arrived. I had spent a very restless night, and even the morphine hadn't been much help when I had tried to fall asleep. As the sun came over the horizon, bright and warm as it shone through my room window, I could feel it on my face, warming me from the inside out. I could feel it's warmth radiating deep down inside, and with a contented sigh I closed my eyes and just enjoyed that warm, fuzzy feeling for several minutes. I was waiting anxiously for my breakfast to arrive, feeling hungry and wondering what they would bring this morning. I hadn't bothered with filling out the menu card the day before that the hospital supplies so we choose our own meals. Although a little tired from not having slept well, I was more excited about getting out of the hospital and going home.

After finishing my breakfast, one of the assistants helped me get dressed in my street clothes. We got all of my things together and put them into my overnight bag and one of the bags supplied by the hospital. I sat there on my bed, all ready to go, but I still had to wait for Dr. Reibel to sign my discharge papers, and the prescriptions to come from the pharmacy. Once I had those then the nurse would arrange for me to get a wheelchair. We had made plans for my brother, Steve, to drive me home, and I wondered what time he would be coming.

Steve has never had any patience waiting around for anything, and today would be no exception. When he walked into the room, he looked as if he expected me to be ready to go and was a little irritated because we had to wait. He paced back and forth and then began flirting with some of the nurses, who seemed to be getting a kick out of this.

One nurse finally brought my discharge papers reviewed the instructions with me, gave me my prescriptions from the pharmacy and stated that transportation was on the way. Steve left the room and went to the garage to get the car, promising to meet me at the main entrance downstairs. On the way home I was feeling hungry and nauseated on my stomach so Steve stopped by McDonalds and bought me an order of fries and a clear soda. I munched on them while he was driving.

Tina had picked Amber up early that morning because they were taking her fishing, and Barbara was outside, sitting at the patio table on the front deck, drinking a cup of coffee when we got there. I was walking very slowly up with sidewalk with Steve holding me up. I hated having to rely on him to help me walk, because it made me feel like a small child being led by the hand. I didn't dare try to balance myself and walk on my own though. So I just let him walk me all the way to the trailer and up those steps, which seemed to be the biggest mountain that I had ever climbed as I made my way up them one at a time.

As we walked into the trailer, I went straight into the living room and settled into the recliner, thankful to be sitting down. Steve explained to Barbara what the doctors and the nurses said were important. He gave her the discharge sheets that had all of the instructions—and dosages of my medicines, and stayed for a very few minutes before driving back home. Mom would probably call and check on me later, he explained. I would first need time to rest for a while.

While it felt so good to be back home (boy had I missed this place I thought, looking around the living room), I felt weak and worn out from that short walk from the car to the house. How long, I wondered, was it going to take for me to regain my strength? Barbara brought me a cool drink and some soup to eat for lunch, since the instructions said that I couldn't take the Roxycet on an empty stomach. She sat on the loveseat and kept me company while I ate. Normally, I would have had the television on, but today, I just wanted to get through eating in peace and quiet. After I finished, Barbara helped me get up out of the chair and into the bedroom. Before lying down, I felt like I had to go to the bathroom, and she helped me walk in there. I stood there for a few minutes but couldn't go, and finally just stretched out in bed to sleep for a while.

When they sedated me to perform the surgery, my bladder had gone to sleep as well. I found it difficult to pass urine from the time that Steve had brought me home. We struggled with walking me back and forth to the bathroom all afternoon after my nap. I would feel the strong urge to go, and Barbara would walk me into the bathroom and stand behind me, with her hands on my waist to hold me up. I would go just a few drops and without warning, it would stop. I would stand there and stand there, but nothing happened. What frustrated me was that as soon as I was sitting back in the recliner, it would hit me again, with the same results.

I was constantly drinking water, milkshakes, tea and even the Ensure to stay hydrated. Liquids were much easier to swallow and actually soothed my irritated throat to some degree. My mouth constantly felt dry and sometimes I would just suck on a piece of candy for the moisture. This went on all day and into the night. I went to bed around 8 that night, exhausted and feeling like I couldn't sit up for another minute. Barbara had to get me up and down several times when my bladder began to hurt from being so full. Finally, I had taken about all of it I could handle. It had been 10 long and frustrating hours, and I knew I was in trouble and needed medical attention. Barbara called 9-1-1, and summoned the rescue squad.

When it's been hours since you've emptied your bladder, every second can seem like it's a day long. I was grouchy and hurting, and the fifteen to twenty minutes that it took for the rescue squad to finally get there seemed like forever. I heaved a huge sigh of relief as we saw the blinking lights when they pulled into our driveway. Barbara unlocked the front door for them to get in.

They brought enough people with them that you would have thought there was a major disaster. They all crowded into our small, cramped living room with their big bags full of the oxygen tanks, blood pressure cuffs and other paraphernalia they used in medical emergencies. When they asked what the problem was, and I explained it to them, they shocked the hell out of me and Barbara. They apologized that I was having such problems but said that it wasn't a medical emergency for them to handle. What! My mouth dropped open and I was left speechless. Not an emergency? Hey, ever had to urinate and can't, I wondered.

Barbara, absolutely furious, told them point blank that if I developed an infection or my body was poisoned because they didn't do their job, she would see they were held personally responsible. That seemed to shake them up a bit, and they said even though it wasn't an emergency, they would be willing to take me in to the emergency room. However, they couldn't guarantee how long it would take to get me there.

One of the members, who didn't look any older than a high school kid, and who had a clipboard in her hand, asked Barbara for a complete list of my medications so that she could write the squad report. Barbara told her to write down: that they had been called, that they came out, that they did absolutely nothing and that they had been asked to leave. That's exactly what happened. In a matter of minutes, Barbara had them packed up and out the door, slamming it none too gently behind the last one walking out.

By the time we got them out of the house and the furniture put back so you could move in the room, it was about one O'clock in the morning. I really needed to go to the hospital because by now I was becoming very nauseated and swelled from the fluid retention. My stomach was very bloated and over top of my pajama bottoms and had sharp pains in it. Barbara went into our bedroom and dialed my mother's number, because at this point it was the only thing that we felt we could do. I couldn't help that it would upset her and she probably wouldn't sleep the rest of the night.

She answered on the fourth ring, and when Barbara explained what was going on, and she heard we'd called the squad and they wouldn't do anything, boy did she curse and get loud enough to wake the dead!

Mom said she would go awaken Steve and he would be there as soon as he could. I knew he was going to definitely have a bad attitude when he got there, because this had interrupted his rest. He works as a logger, often driving distances to job sites, sometimes as far as North Carolina. It's usually late in the evenings when he gets home.

He came in the door in a rush less than an hour later, and wanted to know if I was ready to go. He had to help me get down the steps of the front deck. My legs were weak and it was real tricky for me to walk down them. It never occurred to any of us for me to go out of the back door which had the shorter steps. We had to stop a couple of times for me to rest and catch my breath, before getting to his car at the top of the driveway.

After Barbara called mom, I hadn't bothered to change into street clothes once I knew he was coming to take me to the hospital. I figured it would save physical strength and energy not to have to redo it all again when I got back home. So I just tossed on a light jacket over my pajamas since it was pretty warm outside. It wasn't too muggy and not too chilly. It actually felt pretty good, and the fresh air smelled good. If I hadn't been hurting and feeling so miserable I would have enjoyed it.

When I got to the emergency room, they called me in to the examination room within minutes after I got there. It was better than the time before. They inserted a catheter into my bladder, and drained almost a full quart of urine and then decided since I had had so much trouble, they would leave it in until my bladder started working on its own again.

When the nurse came in with my discharge papers, she also gave me instructions on how to empty and take care of the catheter and told me to come back in four days to have it taken out. I was definitely feeling a lot better by the time Steve got me home about 2 hours later. It was like a "weight" had been removed, and I was able to sleep very well that night. The pain medication might have had something to do with it, since it did contain codeine. But it had sure been a long and active day and I was literally exhausted.

I was not the same man who had left home 4 days earlier, going into the hospital. I was as weak as a day old kitten, and totally dependent on Barbara for simple, basic every day things like bathing, getting dressed, walking, sitting down and getting out of a chair, lying down and getting out of bed, or changing positions while in bed. It was very hard for me to accept. I felt degraded, frustrated, and yes, even angry, being forced to ask her to do all of these things for me. I knew she didn't mind doing it, but it bothered me. I was a grown man, reduced to depending on his wife to dress and undress him like she would a small child.

Barbara spent a lot of time in the kitchen. She was searching through her collection of cookbooks trying to find appetizing foods that I could easily digest and swallow. She was cooking and preparing food and using the small food chopper and blender so I could swallow it. It looked awful and resembled baby food when she finished with it, and not like something I would enjoy one bit. As much as I hated it, I tried not to complain.

She was doing all of the cooking and cleaning, and she logged a lot of steps checking on me, especially if I were lying down in bed. She would bring ice, water, give me all of my medications, come in and help me change positions or to get up to go to the bathroom—anything that I really needed to have done. I think she walked back and forth just to satisfy herself that I was ok, and I called her sometimes when I didn't need a thing—just being tired of being in the room away from everything, by myself.

She gave me a ceramic bell to ring which didn't work out too well because it didn't ring very loud, and sometimes she wouldn't hear it if she were busy washing dishes or was in the other end of the trailer. She finally found a whistle that I could blow—and boy did I use it!

Sometimes I would blow and blow on it until she all but ran to see what I needed, only for me to say "I just wanted to know what you were doing." After a few times doing that she threatened to take it away from me.

Although she never complained out loud, I knew it was hard on her. I would see her sit down on the edge of the bed, pretending she needed to catch her breath, but I knew it was her back that made her sit down. She was trying to hard to keep ahead of everything and I didn't want to make her feel bad so for a while I just watched and kept quiet. But finally, as it became more and more obvious that she was struggling, I couldn't keep my mouth shut any more. I suggested that she call the Orange County Department of Social Services and ask them if they would send out a Home Health Aide. At least they would able to help with some of the work a few times a week which would make it easier on her. Reluctantly she admitted she could use the help and made the call.

I knew she called at my suggestion, and I also knew that she did need the help; but it wasn't really what she wanted to do. She wanted to be the one to take care of me and our home. Ever since we had been together, she had prided herself on being able to keep our home clean and food on the table for me when I came home from work, or from doing the outside chores.

I also knew that when she thought I was asleep she would come to the doorway of the bedroom to look in on me, and she would have tears streaming down her face as she saw me lying there in the bed. It was hard on me being so damned dependent on her—but it was also hard for her, too because she knew how much I wanted to be up and active, but couldn't.

When she made the call, she was left waiting for about five minutes before the person in charge of the program got on the phone. After asking a few background questions, the woman told her that we needed to come in and fill out an application to be screened for services. Barbara explained that she couldn't drive my truck and I had just been discharged from the hospital and was bedridden. The worker scheduled an appointment for early the following week to come out and do an in home interview.

We spent an hour the next week answering question after question like we were revealing our entire life history, which I thought was stupid, just to get a service from them. She finally seemed to be satisfied with the information she had and left, telling us that she would call with her decision by the end of the week.

When Friday went by without hearing anything from her, Barbara called at the end of the day. She was told that we did meet the requirements for the home health aide program, but at the time no one that they had listed in their directory would be willing to drive out to our end of the county to work, and that if we were to find someone who would do the work, and they would be willing to register with their department, then they would pay them.

What? I needed to find someone? How the hell did they expect me to do that when I was lying flat on my back, so weak it was hard to stand up or walk through the floor? And why should I do it anyway? What were they being paid to do?

Barbara, aggravated beyond words, hung the phone up. We decided then and there that we would do the best we could with what we had available and that we wouldn't ask them for any assistance again. Somehow, we managed to get through it although I know we wouldn't have if it had not been for family and friends who pitched in to help us out.

The fourth day of having the catheter in place came, and I would be so glad to have it out. We had made arrangements with a church member, Larry Dudley, to come over after he got home from work to take me back to the emergency room. My bladder, thankfully was working normally, and as many fluids as I was drinking, sometimes a little too well. It seemed as if Barbara constantly had to empty the bag, but hey after what I'd had to deal with, neither one of us was complaining one little bit.

Larry got to the house a little after seven that evening, and Barbara and I were ready and waiting for him. We offered to give him some money for gas since he had to drive from the other side of Fluvanna County, to the hospital, bring us home and then drive back. He refused and said that friends were supposed to help friends when they needed it.

I had about a fifteen minute wait before they took me back into the Nurse Practitioner's Department,(I assumed because it wasn't an emergency, just a routine procedure) where the nurse told me to strip from the waist down and wait for the doctor. The same doctor, (a woman) who had inserted it came in. Without wasting any time, she removed the catheter by giving it a hearty quick pull, practically jerking it out.

OH MY GOD!! Did that ever hurt? I gulped, gasping in pain, a low pain filled groan escaping my lips, as beads of perspiration broke out on my forehead. My God, didn't the woman realize or even give a damn that she could have permanently damaged my bladder not to mention my privates? I lay on the table for several minutes before being able to stand up and get my pants on. It was very painful walking out of there, and standing outside while our friend went to the parking garage to get his car.

The next morning, since the catheter had been removed, I wanted a real bath, not a sponge wash off—but an honest to goodness bath, which I hadn't had since the morning I went into surgery.

I still couldn't get in the shower because of the stitches, but I could certainly sink down into some nice hot water in the big garden tub—and that's exactly what I did. Oh, did it ever feel so good! Barbara helped me bathe and it took a lot of twisting, turning and sweating for me to be able to get out. I had to be careful of my left arm, which was sore and couldn't be tugged.

We were both exhausted by the time I finally had both feet back on the floor. Now, the trick was going to be washing my hair. It really needed it from all of the sweating I had done lying in bed. Since I couldn't get wet from the neck up, Barbara had bought some leave in shampoo in a can. I'd never heard of it, much less tried it. But my hair was starting to itch, so we used it. Well, it wasn't bad I guess, but it didn't feel like it was as clean as it was when I stood under the shower, scrubbing with good smelling shampoo and then rinsing with a great conditioner. The conditioner helped restore body to my hair, which was thin and sort of brittle. But it was better than not doing anything at all.

My brother Michael is the closest one to me in age, and lives the farthest away from the whole family. He lives in Tuscaloosa Alabama and has been down there for years. He has worked in all areas of law enforcement for the past thirty years, and is now talking about retiring sometime in 2008.

He calls my mother every week and always comes in for a visit sometime during the spring or summer each year, and we all look forward to seeing him and catching up with each other. He had planned on coming in early in 2004, but after I was diagnosed with the cancer, and he learned that I would have to have surgery, he postponed his trip to coincide with when the surgery would be done and I was back at home.

Normally, we always drove down to mom's to visit with him while he was here, because after driving all the way through from Alabama to Virginia, the last thing he wanted to do was drive anywhere else. Mom or Steve usually drove him around to visit people in Fluvanna.

At the time I was going through all of the treatments and surgery, he was the Police Chief at the local Veteran's Administration in Tuscaloosa, and took vacation time to come home for a visit.

He and Steve came up to see us at the trailer, and they worked to hook cable up to the little color television that we had in our bedroom. Sometimes, I felt like I wanted to watch television but wasn't up to getting out of bed and going into the living room. He said now I could kick back and watch it all I wanted and relax at the same time.

He sat down in the living room while I ate a snack and had Ensure, and visited with me for over an hour, and it really made me feel good to spend time with him. I really kind of hated to see him leave. He called me several times after that and I managed to talk for a little while. My voice would grow tired and weak after a while, but I just took it slow and had to learn to work around that.

Dependent and Depressed

After my surgery, I was not allowed to drive for almost three months while I recuperated. As unfamiliar as I was at having my freedom restricted like this, it really was a good thing. Most of the things I tried to do, like walking outside in the yard or just sitting for long periods of time, made me stiff, very tired and sleepy.

I was still taking a lot of medication to deal with the pain, and because it upset my stomach, I was also taking anti-nausea medication. This was all new to me and I didn't particularly like it. I'd never been a "pill popper" and only took them when I had to. My doctors didn't go so far as placing a restriction on my license with DMV, but instead trusted that I would take their advice to heart and follow it. Physically I had no choice. Mentally, I was chomping at the proverbial bit. I knew down deep inside they were right, but it didn't mean I had to like it.

I had always been used to going where and when I wanted to. I had learned a long time ago to value my driver's license after being stupid and losing them for a while. It hadn't been any fun having to walk wherever I went or to wait for someone to take me when I needed to go somewhere. Now, having them and not being able to use them was just as frustrating for me.

I had very limited mobility when it came to moving the upper part of my body after the surgery. Steering would have been hard, if not impossible. When they had cut the Sternocleidomastoid muscle to remove the mass, it had made using my left arm almost impossible. It was like a dead weight hanging on that side of my body, and I could barely lift it as high as my waistline. It was also difficult holding light weight things like a fork for any length of time. I've always been left handed in almost everything I do and I actually had to learn how to eat using my right hand. Talk about hard! It was frustrating, messy and sometimes I almost gave up trying to get used to it. I had no measurable range of motion with my neck either. I couldn't turn my head in either direction more than a fraction and even that small amount caused sharp stabbing pains to shoot up the back of my neck.

My days were long, frustrating and very depressing. Sometimes I just felt so despondent that all I wanted to do was stay in bed and not get up unless I had to go to the bathroom, or wanted something to eat. Dr. Reibel refused to let me lay there and wallow in self pity. He was worried that if I stayed in bed without getting exercise, I ran a greater risk of developing pneumonia or other respiratory infections. Any kind of infection would not be a good thing with my compromised immune system. He told Barbara he didn't care how she did it, or how much I fussed and raised hell about it. He wanted me to get up a couple of hours in the morning, a couple in the afternoon and again in the evening.

I couldn't seem to get interested in many of the shows that were on television, although I did watch the news, and every now and then would watch part of a movie. I would cover up with a lightweight quilt, recline my chair back for naps, and eat, drink shakes or whatever else appealed to me at the time. Barbara would be working on things in the house; like cooking, doing dishes, doing the laundry or emptying the trash. As I watched her moving around working, I became even angrier, frustrated and even bitter that she was doing something useful and I was forced to sit in a chair like an old man or invalid and do nothing.

I would sit there thinking about the grass that needed cutting, the outside trash cans that were full and needed go to the dumpster and knowing that there were things we needed from the grocery store. There was a long list of so many things that I needed and wanted to be doing. Damn! When would this ever end so I could feel useful again? It couldn't be soon enough for me.

Barbara's uncle James lived across the road from us. She would sit at the kitchen table and make a list of things she needed, and he would go to the store for her. I know that it aggravated and frustrated her too that she had to depend on him. She really didn't like asking him to do it because she knew that he was in bad shape health wise himself: He was diabetic and took insulin every day, and he had emphysema, which meant that he had to carry oxygen with him every where he went, and he used inhalers and a nebulizer machine like the one she had. He only had thirty percent of his heart functioning, and had suffered a number of heart attacks, and had undergone a by-pass surgery. There were times that he would go to the hospital once or twice a week sometimes for severe chest pains, and a lot of times that they kept him at least overnight. Like a lot of the "old" country folks I knew, he was stubborn and refused to give up. He kept going out of sheer will, determination and grit. Whenever there was work to be done, no matter how bad he felt, or how long it took him he would get it done.

Sandy and one the guys who helped her around the church came over and drove Barbara to Food Lion when she needed to do a lot of grocery shopping. They helped her bring everything inside so that she could get it put it away. They came into the living room to pray for me and then they left to go back to Charlottesville. My sister Linda came to visit one day and we needed a few odds and ends so Linda drove her to Food Lion and brought her home before leaving. June came up early one morning and took me once I was up on my feet enough to move around. By then I had gone to the pharmacy and bought a cane which helped me on weak days, and gave me more stability.

I still felt like I wasn't doing enough, and that it was all too much for Barbara. I had finally gotten to the point that I could move around a little, and sometimes I would take the kitchen trash outside to the can, or other little small chores. A lot of the time I felt depressed, like I was on what Tommy used to call "a pity party." I couldn't do what I enjoyed and was used to taking care of myself, not being waited on by anybody else.

I hated it when the grass got tall enough and I knew that my brother-in-law was driving up from his house to cut it. I did appreciate that he did it for me, that wasn't the problem. It was just that it really irked me that he had to cut the grass, and all I could do was sit helplessly out on the front deck under the shade of the umbrella and watch. I wanted to be the one out there in the yard, riding up and down and seeing how good it looked as I worked on cutting it.

Our landlord can be a real pain in the neck sometimes and he stopped by the house once when I first came home from the hospital, and the grass was getting tall and needed to be cut. It was early in the week and Harold hadn't had time to get up here to cut it. The landlord knocked on the front door, and when Barbara answered it, he told her that the grass had to be cut and if we didn't get to it in a couple of days, he would cut it and charge us $40.00. Barbara exploded.

She told him that I was bedridden from just having my throat opened to remove throat cancer, and with taking care of me and the way her back was she couldn't do it, and that it was that important to her; but for him to go ahead and cut it and try to charge her for it and she would have his ass in court so fast his head would fly off his shoulders. He didn't cut the grass. He never came back to complain about it. And it got cut when Harold could get to it.

Not everything during this time was so boring, frustrating or bad. I know you are wondering if we ever had any happy moments during all of this. Yes. We did. Unfortunately, when everything in your life has been completely turned upside down, they are few and far between.

There were a couple of events that happened during this time that helped revive my sagging spirits and made me feel good. The best part was that they actually got me out and away from the house for a change, and to me that was the best part of all. For Barbara, I think it was just a relief to finally be able to take a break from doing housework and getting to sit down and rest and enjoy being around people for a change.

My mother's birthday is September 17, and because it was on a weekday this year, my sister Darlene decided to have the celebration the weekend afterwards. She put together a cookout and party to celebrate my mother's 75th birthday, and my coming through my cancer surgery. I was still on the driving restriction, and my sister Linda drove us down to the cookout. I put my window down, and Ahhh!! Everything looked so green and alive, and the breeze blowing into the car smelled so fresh.

We talked, laughed and joked around with each other as Linda drove us to the country. It seemed that we never got together with each other anymore unless it was at holidays or if someone in the family died. It was like we were all rushing through our own lives, and never took time to share it with each other. She had gotten new dentures, and she was telling us how many problems she was having with them, and I was really surprised that she thought part of it was funny. I had no idea that day that several months down the road I would be dealing with dentures myself.

When we got to Darlene's there was a small crowd of people already there, and some of them Barbara and I hadn't seen for a long time. My mother was sitting on the deck talking to Helen Johnson and when I walked up onto the deck, she hugged me and gave me a big kiss on my cheek. Maybe any other time it would have embarrassed me. I hugged and kissed her back, and she didn't complain when I squeezed a little too hard, just a soft grunt of protest. Looking around, I noticed the banners that Darlene had hung up. One said "Happy Birthday" and the one under it said "Congratulations." It really meant a lot that the cookout was for me and mom. I was hungry for food and hoped that there was some I wouldn't have much problem eating.

I sat outside on the deck for a while talking to everyone who stopped to speak to me and finally made my way inside the house to go to the bathroom. Darlene had all of the food sitting on the table and on the countertops in the kitchen, and boy did it ever smell and look delicious. If it hadn't been for the dry mouth from the radiation my mouth would definitely have been watering as I took it all in.

I wanted to walk for a bit and left the deck to walk around and look at all of the remodeling Harold and Darlene had had done to their house. It really looked good. The big back deck and the front one with the roof over top of it made me a little envious. I wished I had one to enjoy. Their youngest son Jason was sitting on the porch chilling out with one of his friends, so I stopped and talked to him for a few minutes.

Everyone enjoyed good food and drinks and lots of laughter. It was a good day celebrating as a family. I sat there watching it all, saying a silent prayer of thanks that everything had turned out good for me and I gave thanks that I was able to sit here and enjoy friends and family on such a beautiful crisp afternoon.

For me to be able to get out of the house had me feeling like I had this depression thing licked, at least for the day. I'd worry about tomorrow when it got here. One thing I had learned from all of this was not to rush one minute of the time God granted me to be on this earth. But it was hard.

When you are forced to go from being able to work and earn a paycheck, drive where you want to go, do the chores and hobbies that you enjoy and that need to be done, and are active to being totally dependent on the government, other people, have to struggle to eat, rely on one medication after the other it is hard. You want everything to hurry up, get back to normal. Unfortunately, the "normal" I had known in the past was gone. I would have to find my own "new normal", and it would be a long and frustrating search.

TEST AND MEND

Six weeks after I was released from the hospital, I was scheduled for my first visit with Dr. Reibel to see how the surgical site was healing. I admit I was feeling more than a little apprehensive and nervous as I walked through the door of the clinic. But I shook my head and was determined that I wasn't going to borrow trouble or jump to conclusions and would just wait to see what he had to say when I saw him.

His office on Fontaine Avenue in the new Research Park was very nice and had a "friendly" sort of atmosphere. It wasn't stuffy and institutional like most of the ones at the main hospital. The furniture reminded me of being in a den or small living room, and there was a television for patients to enjoy while they waited. All of the nurses and staff were friendly and welcoming, with warm greetings when I checked in.

One nurse in particular I had taken an instant liking to was Ellen Desper. She was outgoing, honest and friendly, and very competent. She always took extra time to listen to how I felt or about any problem I was having, and then tried to help solve it. I wondered how she found so much energy every day. Every time I had been to the clinic the waiting room was full of patients, so she must stay busy for the most part of it.

Ellen called me into the back and the first thing she did was do a weight check. I knew I had lost more weight because my jeans didn't fit well any more and I'd had to put more holes in my belt, after going down a couple of sizes on the jeans. If I didn't start gaining some weight, or at least stop losing so much pretty soon I'd have to find a way to buy new jeans because I was running out of ones that fit right.

It wasn't that I didn't eat, I did. I ate; I drank the Ensure and milkshakes, but for some reason my weight just kept going down instead of up. After doing a quick temperature and blood pressure check, Ellen said Dr. Reibel would be in shortly, and closed the door as she stepped out

Within a few minutes, Dr. Reibel came bouncing into the room, with his black patent shoes clicking on the tile floor. It reminded me of a woman wearing high heels. Slinging his long lab coat out of the way, he plopped down on the round wheeled stool close to the chair I was sitting in and asked me how I was feeling. He still hadn't managed to make eye contact with me because he was busy looking at notes in my chart

He finally closed it, and gave it a toss to send it sliding across the countertop. He proceeded to feel of my neck with his hands, moving rapidly up and down, and turning my head side to side. Reaching over into a tall glass cylinder he pulled out one of the extra-long tongue blades. He told me to open wide, and say ahhhh. Uhh, damn I thought, this sucks, as I felt my gag reflex being pressed as he glanced down my throat. I closed my eyes and started counting to ten to relax. Finally satisfied, he slowly withdrew it and tossed it into the trash can.

He told me that everything was looking pretty good, and asked me if I was able to move my arm head and neck without pain or stiffness.

When I told him not very well, he suggested that I speak with Larry Haywood before leaving the clinic. He wrote me a refill for the Roxycet in case I needed it and said that he wanted to see me back in one month for another check up. Larry Haywood, I remember thinking. Who is that? I walked out of the examination room perplexed. The name did sound a little familiar but I was having trouble placing it. I had been introduced to so many people since all of this began, pretty soon all of the names and faces became one big blur.

It turned out that Larry was a volunteer in the clinic, and was a cancer survivor himself. He had been diagnosed with cancer on both sides of his throat and had undergone a bilateral (or double) neck dissection, Chemotherapy and radiation treatment when they used Cobalt 60, before it was discontinued. It showed how ignorant I was because I had no clue what the difference between Cobalt 60 and the radiation I had gone through was.

To look at Larry you would never guess that he is a cancer survivor. He's about six foot three and weighs about two hundred and fifty pounds, with a shaved head and a long, thick, pointed mustache and goatee.

Having experienced the same mobility problems I was now dealing with, he and his wife Tona had developed an exercise program designed specifically to strengthen the shoulder and restoring a greater mobility. Today, Larry travels all across the United States, teaching the program to hospitals and clinics who want to use it in their rehabilitation programs.

When I walked out of the examination room, I wasn't in the mood to talk to a volunteer about some stupid program. All I wanted to do was go home and get something to eat, tell Barbara what the doctor had said, and relax. Larry approached me as I was waiting for the receptionist to print out my next appointment. He had in his hand a video, and was explaining the exercises to me.

I had my black cowboy hat in my hand, and was wearing a black western shirt with gold piping on the pockets and my initialed belt and bolo tie, and black suede cowboy boots. I don't know why, but I always liked to dress in this outfit when I went to the doctor. Maybe it was because it made me feel good about myself, normal again, and gave me the confidence to get through the appointment.

I told Larry straight up I wasn't interested in the video and didn't want to do it. He looked me straight in the eye and I'll never forget what he said to me. It helped to turn things around for me. He said "Well, don't take the damn tape then. But don't come in six months from now bitching, moaning and groaning because you still can't use your arm".

It shocked me speechless, and I didn't say anything for a few seconds. I couldn't believe that he had actually said that to me just because I had said that I wasn't interested in the video he had in his hand. Then I remembered that Dr. Reibel had asked me to talk to Larry before I left. I held my hand out and said, "Give me the tape." He handed it to me and said he'd trade me my hat for the tape, and we both laughed. Barbara had gone with me that day, and she still tells Larry to this day that she is so glad he took that attitude with me because it made all the difference in the world.

It was several days before I got the nerve up to pop the video tape into the VCR to see what I would have to do with this rehabilitation program of Larry's. Well, it looks simple enough, I remember saying to Barbara as we sat in our living room watching it together. HA! I just thought it was simple! None of the exercises looked complicated at all.

Once I started doing the exercises, it didn't take me long to realize that it was going to be a long, slow and very painful program. There were days I was sore and achy and just didn't do them, but for the most part I tried to do them every morning or afternoon, and sometimes both.

It did eventually pay off, and today I'm thankful for it because I have greater mobility and use of my arm again, but of course, I still deal with stiffness and joint pain on a daily basis.

An Unexpected Tragedy

December 3, 2004 was just an ordinary day, and dawned like any other winter morning, cold. It might warm up when the sun came out. Barbara and I slept late that morning, and then after breakfast headed out to the bank to pay bills and then on to the grocery store to pick up what we really needed before going back home.

For the most part we stayed around the house that day. After putting away the groceries and fixing supper, Barbara drew a tub of hot water to soak in for a while, and I sat down to watch the news. Sometimes we would pop a bowl of popcorn or take some fruit into the back bedroom we had made into a den, and sit to watch television, and still be able to see who was coming in and out of the trailer park, since the window faced the entrance to the main road.

After her bath, Barbara fixed each of us a plate of cheese and crackers and we sat down to watch a movie on television. About 8:30, the telephone rang, causing Barbara to have to lower her footrest on the recliner and get up to cross the room to answer it. It was not a call we were expecting to get.

It was Peggy Douglas on the other end, and she wanted to know if anybody had called to let us know how Jason was doing. We were totally confused. Jason? What was wrong with Jason? Jason was my sister Darlene's youngest son, and as far as we knew he was fine.

According to Peggy, he had been in a bad wreck earlier and Joey, my brother Steve's son had been in the car with him.

Barbara managed to thank her for calling and hung up the phone to tell me. It hit me hard. All I could think was I should get up and get dressed so we could drive over to the hospital. I cried and was shaking like a leaf.

I was still having a hard time accepting the fact that Jason had been in a wreck. When we had been at Darlene's for the cookout, Jason and some of his friends were hanging out on the front porch of the house, and driving up and down the road in his car. I spent some time talking to him and he seemed happy and care-free, just the way he always did.

Jason had picked Joey up from his house on Route 631 (Bybee Church Road). At a little after 7, Jason lost control of his car and hit a big oak tree directly across from Bybee Road Church. They transported Jason by Pegasus and Joey by ambulance to UVa Hospital. Steve, Darlene, Harold and mom were over there. We were going to go over there, but then decided there wasn't any point that night and that we would wait until the next morning.

We turned off the television and held each other and prayed that Jason and Joey would be alright and asked Him to bless the doctors who were working on them, to guide them as they used all of their medical knowledge to heal whatever was wrong. It was a long night for both of us and I don't think either of us got more than an hour or two of sleep.

We went to the hospital the next morning and the waiting room was full of people waiting for news. Both of them had been taken to the Intensive Care Unit with extensive injuries, and Darlene and Harold looked very lost and upset as they sat there. It was touch and go for both of them for quite some time. I did go in to see Jason, and tears welled in my eyes as I saw him lying there with all of the machines. I kissed his hand and told him to hurry and get well.

Jason was outgoing, friendly with a great sense of humor and a personality that drew people to him. He made friends everywhere he went. He loved sports, especially little league and baseball. Darlene drove him all over the state every year to play in tournaments and he was a good player. Another one of his passions was hunting. He went hunting every year with his dad Harold and his brother Brian. They would even hunt on Thanksgiving Day, coming out of the mountains long enough to come by moms to eat dinner before going back again.

The doctors tried valiantly, with everything that they knew to correct the injuries that Jason suffered in the wreck. There was only so much that they could do, and he was placed on a ventilator that would breathe for him. On December 16th, Darlene and Harold were faced with a decision that no parent, under any circumstance, wants to be forced to make.

After extensive testing on his brain function failed to show any sign of improvement, the family gathered in Jason's room to say goodbye. Then everyone left the room except for Darlene and Harold.

They made the heart-breaking decision to disconnect the ventilator and let Jason go on to Heaven, where he would be at peace and not suffer any pain. It's something no one in this family will ever forget. The tears and pain of losing your child, especially so tragically and at such a young age is something you carry with you until your dying breath.

Out of respect for his family and his friends and all who knew him, the family left his casket closed at family night and during the beautiful graveside service. He was laid to rest beside his grandfather on December 20, 2004, but he will always been missed and never forgotten.

Joey had also received severe and life-threatening injuries in the wreck and that was what made all of it even harder for the family to deal with. He had to go through several surgeries to repair the injuries he had received, and it was touch and go for quite some time with him. The family alternated between spending time with both of them, all of us leaning on each other for support to get through it.

The doctors were concerned that some of the injuries that Joey had suffered would prevent him from walking again once he healed. But, like all of the Moore family, Joey is a fighter and a survivor, and through grit, determination and rehabilitation, has proved them wrong.

I had my church praying for them both, and they were kept on the prayer list daily. I had a hard time dealing with it, and even though I was going through a hell of my own, somehow I didn't feel that it even came close to what everyone else was dealing with right then.

Since that time Joey has taken photography classes and has become quite an accomplished photographer in his own right. He takes detailed pictures that most people would overlook, or just not think worthy of photographing. A few of his pictures have won awards, and all of the family is very proud of him for doing something he likes and doing it so well.

Revs Up the Sun

Barbara's Cousin Tammy lived in Greene County and they talked off and one at least once or twice a month. One afternoon she called Barbara and read her a classified ad in our local paper. It was about a woman who designed rooms for people who were cancer patients. It was called "Rooms for a Reason" and it sounded interesting to Barbara. Tammy read her off the number and she wrote it down, and told Tammy she would call later that night to find out more information and let her know about it the next day.

When she first telephoned all she got was a recording and so she left her name and number and waited for someone to call her back. Kathy Lindstrom it turned out was a cancer survivor herself. She had been treated for breast cancer with the same treatments I was getting. Barbara briefly outlined what I had gone through, and she wrote down the information, my name and address and made an appointment to come out a couple of days later to meet us and to look at the trailer.

She was a petite woman, with bright blue eyes, a nice friendly smile and short blonde hair that looked wind-blown. The style of the cut really looked good on her. We all sat at the kitchen table and she asked questions about my type of cancer, the treatments I'd taken, and what my prognosis was.

She told us that after her husband had redone their bedroom, making her a place to unwind and relax after going through chemotherapy, she thought all cancer patients should be so lucky. It was why she had started her little business. She told us with her small budget, all she could afford were small things, and anything large would depend on the public being generous with donations.

Our trailer was a 2001 model from Clayton Homes and it didn't need anything done to it structurally. After doing a walk-through, Kathy sat down and asked me questions like what I liked to do and some of the hobbies I enjoyed. Being from country, I really liked being outside, especially fishing and puttering around in the yard.

Because of radiation and being limited to time out in the sun, I still wanted to be outside, so what I really wanted done was for her to build me a front deck onto the trailer. We had a small stoop at both the front and the back doors. The front porch we very seldom used because the steps were long and steep, and it was hard for Barbara to climb them, and now, since I was weak and got tired so easily, I didn't use them very often either. She said she would see what she could up with as far as materials to put up a small deck.

The first thing we had to do before Kathy could go any further with her plans was to get permission from our landlord, Bill Willard, because we didn't own the property. We really didn't like to have to call him for anything, and about the only time we ever saw any of them was when they picked up the check for our lot rent at the end of each month. When Barbara called him, he said that he would stop by so we could show him what we wanted to do. A couple of days later he came by and after we told him what we wanted and who would be doing the work, he said that he had no problem with it as long as the work, when it was finished, met the building codes for Orange County.

It took several weeks for Kathy to get all of the materials she needed for building the deck, but it was the following weekend when she, her husband and two friends who helped out, arrived to get started on a plan they had for the inside. They had found me a nice dresser that I needed for my clothes and they had discussed putting up shelves to hold my wife's bric a brac and it just so happened that we had two that June had given us when we had been down to her house. Kathy had taken them with her and had them painted to match the curtains and wallpaper in our bedroom and bathroom.

They hung one in the bedroom for my wife's ceramic bell collection, some of which had belonged to her mother, and the other one they put in our bathroom for toiletries or small items. The dresser looked antique in style and had a large mirror attached to it which we both liked. The only full length mirror we had was the one behind the garden tub in our bathroom.

I had also told Kathy that I was a big sports fan, especially UVA and NASCAR. Between Barbara and me we had a small collection of Earnhardt memorabilia. The back bedroom (that is now my wife's office) was my den—that we had haphazardly put together with two recliners, and the television which had been Barbara's mother's. The television and our VCR were sitting on a small wooden television stand. We didn't use the room much at the time and hadn't had time to put it together in a better way. Kathy and her team completely redid the entire room.

We had a large wall unit entertainment center from Wal-Mart, for the new color television we'd bought at Schewel Furniture Company when we furnished the trailer. After I spent hours trying to put the thing together it was wobbly, and to get it to stand straight, I had to attach it to the wall with the straps that were stapled onto the back of it. It turned out that the television we had bought was too tall to fit on it, and I had put it in our bedroom. We had a small color television, some whatknots and a lot of books and other junk scattered on it.

Kathy and her "team" cleaned everything off of it and moved it from our bedroom into the den. They put the television and VCR on it, along with all of our Earnhardt collection. They hung the pictures, portraits and large throws on the walls, and put new curtains on the windows. We were very impressed because they had it looking a lot homier and a lot more comfortable than it had been, and it was definitely a man's room.

About a week later, a crew of men spent about four days building a 10"x10" deck. Kathy went to Wal-Mart and bought a patio set for it, with a glass table, umbrella and four patio chairs. She gave us a large planter full of herbs she had planted for us and a large Dale Earnhardt racing flag with a steel pole to hang on the front of the deck. I really enjoyed sitting outside on cool evenings

We called Tammy back to thank her for thinking of us when she had read the advertisement in the paper and for her to come down and see what Rooms for a Reason had done for us. Without her, none of it would have been possible.

Seeking Support

From the time I was first diagnosed with the cancer, almost everyone around me, from Dr. Reibel, Dr. Read, Vikki Bravo and almost every member of my family and most of my friends, kept talking to me about support groups. They suggested that I needed to find out where one was held and go to the meeting. I needed to be around people who knew all about cancer, blah blah blah. They told me that these people could offer moral support, suggestions for problems I was having, this and that and everything in between. Deep down inside I knew that they were right, and yeah, even that I could have used people like that. I just didn't want to hear about it. Sometimes felt like I would scream if I heard just one more word about a group.

I knew that they all loved me and that they were just trying to help. It was their way of trying to be involved in what I was dealing with, but I was too blind to see it at the time. But for me, sitting in a room surrounded by strangers and telling them personal details of the things I was going through, wasn't something that I felt like I was ready to do at the time. I didn't rule it out all together, though. Maybe when things settled down I would think about it then. I just didn't want people to think that they could keep bugging me until I gave in and went to please them.

The major problem in this area that I was having was the fact that I still hadn't come to terms with everything in my life that had been affected by cancer: the way I was having to eat, my sleep patterns had been changed, being active—or I should say not being able to be active enough, and even my sex life was limited. I was taking more medication than I wanted to: medications for this problem, that side effect and the other, as well as over-the-counter stuff. I still had the stomach tube dangling uselessly from my stomach. Dr. Reibel hadn't decided to take out yet, even if the number of times I'd used it could be counted on one hand. Since I hadn't learned how to accept it, why should people who didn't know me from Adam be worried about what I thought and felt? Forget it! I didn't want to hear any more about a support group.

I had so much on my plate that to this day I'm not sure how I kept it all straight. I wouldn't have been able to if Barbara wasn't such a good organizer. She kept my medication doses on schedule; the refills always ready to be picked up when they had to be refilled, and my appointments marked clearly on the calendar so I could read them. Speaking of appointments, I was going back and forth to so many different clinics and treatments, that they should have given me my own permanent parking spot! Support groups on top of all of this? Bah! Forget it!

Vikki Bravo, in addition to be a social worker in the cancer center was also the facilitator of the support group, who focused on the people who had been diagnosed with oral, head and neck cancer at the hospital. Although I hadn't taken her up on her suggestion to come to a meeting, she had put my name on the group's mailing list so that I got a newsletter each month. It contained news from the previous meeting, upcoming events and when the next meeting was going to be held. Barbara always read it and would drop subtle hints which I stubbornly ignored; so she would leave it lying on the kitchen table. I really liked Vikki and appreciated her wanting to help me. She reminded me quite often of the energizer bunny as she moved rapidly from one part of the cancer center to the other. She always had a smile on her face and a kind word or hug for those she met.

Now, with the chemotherapy, radiation and the surgery behind me, I felt like I could think more clearly. I thought that I was ready to finally move on to something else. One morning after breakfast, I shocked Barbara by picking up the latest newsletter and sitting down to read it as I finished a cup of coffee. After finishing the newsletter, I told her that I was thinking about going to the meeting that was scheduled for the next day. I didn't want to go by myself though, and asked her if she would mind going with me. I think that she was glad that I had finally come to my senses, so she didn't hesitate and agreed to go.

I had never been to any kind of support group before and had no idea how they worked or what to expect. When we got to the meeting the next day, I hesitated before walking into the room because I was nervous and more than a little apprehensive. A large group of people were sitting around a long conference table. Vikki jumped up from her chair, coming over to hug us. She said she was so glad we were there. There was food for lunch that had been provided by a local restaurant near the "corner" (as everything around the University was called), and she told us to help ourselves to all we wanted.

I introduced myself and Barbara, saying I preferred to listen and not participate. And it didn't seem to bother anyone that I wasn't ready to share. Everyone was courteous, friendly, and I watched in silence as they teased and joked among themselves like they had known each other all of their lives. They had certainly opened up their ranks and made myself and Barbara feel right at home. It wasn't as bad as I had thought it was going to be. Maybe I could get something out of this after all. I mean, it was only once a month, right?

As the meeting closed, Vikki said to me that she was delighted that I had finally quit being so stubborn and decided to join them, and that she hoped we would come back for the meeting next month. Barbara and I have been an active part of that little group of "extended family" ever since, and have only missed three meetings. Whenever we don't go to one we actually miss seeing the group members. We've become very good friends with most of them and they really are like part of my family. We share all kinds of things that help each other, and just to sit around and spend that hour together means a lot; even if we don't do anything more than just share lunch.

In May 2006, Second Wind, our little support group, celebrated their 10th anniversary with a gathering of survivors, caregivers, patients and staff from all areas of the Cancer Center. It was held in Jordan Hall at the University. I estimate there was close to 200 people who came out that day to enjoy the delicious food and drinks. They shared their thoughts and feelings with each other and listened to great speeches by several keynote speakers.

Sadly, I attended the celebration alone, because Barbara was sick with a severe case of bronchitis and didn't feel up to going out of the house. I know that she would have thoroughly enjoyed some of the guest speakers and what they had to share about their cancer experiences and some of the things that they had discovered on their journey. One of the special things was that all of the group members and their spouses stopped long enough to pose for a group picture together, and Vikki made sure that all of us got our own copy to keep as a memento. For now, mine is in one of our photo albums, but I am planning on buying a nice frame for it and then hang it in our living room. I'm proud of it, and each one of the people that are in it with me.

Strive to Survive

The yard sale that we held with our church, when they donated the things from their storage shed to us, had been something that we had not really expected to have a great deal of success with. At first, after setting up our part of the sale, we had the idea that people were buying from us for the simple reason that we were set up on the church property, and they somehow felt obligated to buy a little something so they wouldn't hurt our feelings. We quickly learned that we had assumed wrong as the sale continued.

As they shopped, the people were genuinely interested to learn that I was fighting cancer and still found the energy to get out and earn the money we needed. I suppose a lot of people would have sat around their house and waited for some organization to come along and offer them a hand out or a quick solution to their problems. Well, that just wasn't me, and Barbara wouldn't have gone along with it either. Like myself, she had grown up in the country and although they didn't have a lot, her family worked for what they did have and took care of it.

I wasn't fond of doing the yard sales, but I was not about to sit on my backside and have people hand me what I needed, or considering me a charity case either. I have had countless people since those days tell me that they have no idea how in the world I manage to do what I did to put those sales out. I can't give you an answer to that either, except to say that God gave me the strength to do what I needed to do. It was definitely hard work. The sales we did weren't like the ones people have at their house where they would sit out a couple of tables and put the stuff out, and take it in at the end of the day. If only it had been that simple.

I stacked and lifted totes, boxes and trash bags full of stuff and it was like putting a giant jigsaw puzzle together. There was a certain way that it all had to stack on top of each other on the bed of my truck, so that it could be tied down with rope and bungee cords, so we wouldn't lose anything as I was driving down the road. The distance would depend on where we were holding that particular sale.

When Barbara first came up with her idea of advertising in the Blue Ridge Buck Saver, I was against it. It was a local bi-weekly publication where people could advertise items for sale, items wanted, yard sales, etc.; How would it be successful, who would donate, would it be worth it? I had a lot of questions, but never having done anything like it, I had no answers. So after much discussion, we decided it couldn't hurt to give it a try.

We sat down and wrote out how we thought the ad would grab readers attention, and came up with "Wanted: any usable household item in good condition for a benefit yard sale, to help a cancer patient pay for medical bills and expenses. If you would like to donate, please call ***-***-****. (Phone number hidden for privacy) We will pick up any donations." When we agreed it sounded good, Barbara called the free ad-taker line in Crozet, Virginia and placed the ad for the next publication, due out the following week.

We wondered how it would be received. We thought maybe we would get a call or two for small items. At the time we put that first ad in the paper, we had absolutely no idea that it would take off like a rocket ship and that it would consume a lot of our time and energy for the next couple of years.

The first week our ad was in circulation we only got one or two calls. The items were in ok condition once we took the time to get them cleaned up. Shortly after that we began to get calls for everything ranging from clothing of all kinds and sizes, to furniture, outside toys and appliances. A lot of the calls were from people who lived here in the Barboursville area or maybe just outside, in Albemarle County; so it didn't take much gas or time for us to pick it up.

As time went on and our ad stayed in the paper, we eventually began receiving calls from gated communities, and well-to-do-neighbor-hoods and a lot of the stuff that the people were donating were brand spanking new, some with the price tags still on them. What we had thought would be small yard sales had suddenly and quickly ballooned into flea market sized ones. We were scrambling and racking our brains trying to come up with ideas of where on earth to hold sales this large. Sandy, once again came to our rescue. Living Stones always did so well with the sales they held at the church. It was in a central location and she offered to let us set them up there. She also loaned us the tables from downstairs in the Fellowship Hall, and believe me, with the quantity of stuff we were picking up every week, we took advantage of every square inch of them and the church yard.

We had the tables set out all the way across the yard; we had stuff hanging on borrowed clothes racks; we had big heavy items sitting all the way down the sidewalk; and we had pictures and posters leaning against the rock wall with the Church name and service information on it.

When we held the first sale, people were walking around browsing and trying to buy items before we ever opened the sale, and while we were still unloading items from the boxes and totes to set them out on the tables. We hadn't had the time to make or put out any signs around the area to advertise the sale, but from the looks of it we didn't need to. It seemed like the system known as word of mouth was working just fine. People who lived within a 10 mile area of the church were showing up.

The amount of clothing that people had donated to us was overwhelming to say the least. It allowed us to sell clothing at almost give away prices. We had the Food Lion grocery bags that we let people stuff for one dollar; the white 13 gallon bags they could stuff for three dollars; and the 33 gallon bags they could stuff for five dollars. The expensive or new clothing went onto the racks and ranged from one dollar up to twenty dollars each, and even they moved at a surprising rate.

To save space on the table for dishes and other smaller items that should be displayed on flat surfaces, we put down large blue tarps on the ground and then dumped the every day clothing out onto them. We had women and some men, actually sitting down in the middle of those piles of clothing, and slinging them from side to side as they stuffed the bags. If only I had had a camera back then! I could have sold the pictures to a newspaper or Ripley's Believe it or Not and made a lot of money. Some people just love yard sales and certainly didn't mind doing what it took to find bargains at them. It was hilariously funny at times.

We held the first yard sale from Wednesday thru noon on Saturday and were absolutely shocked when we counted the profits. We had cleared over $500 after taking out what we had spent on gas, drinks and food for the week.

I am not going to say it was amazing or that we did anything that caused us to have a great success. I give God all the credit for what happened in the church yard that week. The first thing we did before opening the sale each morning was to hold hands and pray. We always prayed and thanked God for watching over us and guiding us through the day when we closed it up in the evenings. Now, as we prepared to close the sale for the final time that week, and pack it up and go home, we prayed again, thanking Him and praising Him for everything He'd done for us all during the week.

As time went on and we continued getting calls to pick up donations, we often found ourselves stunned at the amount of stuff people either accumulated or just wanted to get rid of. Sometimes a caller would tell us over the telephone when they called that they had a few items they wanted to donate. When we got to their house, we found that it was an entire truckload. Every now and then we would run across a pick up where most of it was junk and not worth the time we had taken to go get it, and we would have to take it to the county landfill. During the entire time we held the sales we may have made three trips to the landfill, which wasn't a bad ratio considering the amount of stuff we picked up.

Some of the items we had in abundance were clothing, microwaves, televisions, toys, stuffed animals, shoes and books. All of our items sold very well. We always tried to be reasonable in the way we priced them. People were kind enough to donate to us and we weren't trying to get rich off of it. Our main goal was to pay our bills and be able to buy food and things that we really needed. Barbara was always willing to negotiate when someone really wanted something and didn't have enough money. There were also times that she gave quite a bit away to the elderly or people she knew didn't have much money.

We picked up donations from Charlottesville, Scottsville, Earlysville, Louisa, Greene County, Amherst County and Nelson County. Sometimes people would call us more than once to give us stuff and we had quite a few regulars who called us year after year. Some of them, knowing my limitations with my shoulder, would actually help us load and tie the stuff in too.

One time our stock had become low because we hit a dry spell where we weren't getting calls for pick ups. Barbara came up with what I thought at first was a stupid idea. We always read the paper to make sure our ad was listed and that it was worded right, and then looked to see how many yard sales were in the area for that week. Barbara's idea was to call the people who had the ads listed and were having sales.

She thought that maybe they might be willing to donate whatever leftovers they had at the end of their sale. A lot of people, once they finished a sale didn't want to have to worry with packing everything up or finding a place to store it again until they could have another one. Sometimes, that was the only one they were planning to have that year. I went along with it but didn't think that it would amount to anything worthwhile.

Over the next several weeks Barbara would check out the paper each time it came out and place several calls for any sales that looked promising. Sometimes she would only get an answering machine, but not to be outdone, she would leave her name, phone number and why she was calling and then wait to see if she got a response. One such response stands out vividly in my mind, and was a total shock to both of us.

A local family who lived in Charlottesville had advertised that they were having a large moving sale for an entire week. Barbara thought that it would be a good one to call and ask because it could be a lot of good stuff. She figured if they had anything left and were moving, they might donate it to us just so they wouldn't have to deal with it or have to move it twice. She called and left our name and number on their answering machine, and being busy with different things all week, forgot all about it.

The weather that entire week was stormy and we had thunderstorms and rain almost every day, and a downpour on Saturday. We got up early on Sunday morning and had a light breakfast and drank coffee before getting dressed to go to church. The telephone rang as we were heading out, and Barbara, out of habit and thinking that it could be important, walked back into the living room to answer it. I followed her inside in time to see her fall down into the chair at her computer with a shocked look on her face.

Barbara covered the mouthpiece of the phone and told me that it was the lady who had advertised the moving sale. She thanked her for calling us back and then asked how successful her sale had been. The woman said because it had rained the whole week they had decided not to have it and she was calling to find out if we were still interested in the stuff that they had been going to sell. Barbara answered yes immediately, and then asked if it would be alright if we came by and picked it up after we left church services.

The lady asked her what kind of truck we had, and when Barbara said it was a Chevy S-10, the lady laughed and said that it would take several truckloads if we were going to get it all. The problem, she went on to explain to Barbara, was that it all had to be moved out of the house by five O'clock that very afternoon. Shocked, Barbara quickly recovered and asked the lady if it would be alright to call her back in a few minutes to let her know what time we would be there. Thanking her again, she hung up the phone, and gave me a dumbfounded look. Then she said, "Dwayne, a whole house full!"

She went into the kitchen to grab a cigarette and another cup of coffee before dialing Sandy's cell phone number. She wanted to explain to her why we weren't going to be at church this morning so that she wouldn't worry and think something was wrong. When she failed to get an answer on Sandy's cell phone or at the church, she hung up and called her friend, June Dudley.

When June answered the phone, Barbara asked her to tell Sandy that we wouldn't be at church because we had gotten a call to pick up a house full of stuff a woman was donating for our sales, and that we had until that evening to get it out. June was shocked, and wanted to know how we were going to manage that by ourselves. Barbara told her that she honestly didn't know but we would do the best we could with it. June asked her to hold on for a minute while she went to find her husband Jerry to ask him a question.

When she came back on the line she said that she had to ask Jerry if it was ok first because they had a meeting for the motorcycle club after church today and she usually kept notes and things for him. She said that she would use her truck and help us pick all of it up and that she would meet us at the church. June at that time was helping to collect stuff for a new outreach program the church was starting. It was called Transitional Housing and the way it worked was the church would rent houses and furnish them, and then rent rooms out to people who were being released from Prison and drug rehabilitation programs in an effort to help them make a fresh start. June was hoping that there was stuff being donated that maybe they could use for the program.

We knew from the telephone call that none of the stuff had been packed. The lady said that a lot of it was sitting on tables down in the basement and that we would have to bring boxes and newspapers so that the glassware wouldn't be broken or damaged. We wondered just how much stuff we were talking about as we drove into Charlottesville to the church. When the three of us followed her into the basement, our mouths dropped open as our eyes took in all of the stuff down there.

There was over 3 large tables full of dishes: everything from good quality china and crystal, to set after set of dinnerware, silverware, wine goblets, Japanese tea sets, what knots, games, computer parts, adding machines, crocheted spreads, afghans, brand name clothing, shoes, a queen-size futon (with cover), laundry hampers, quilts, bric-a-brac, artificial plants, Christmas trees, holiday decorations—the list seemed endless. Everywhere we looked we saw stuff that would have to be bagged or packed into cardboard boxes.

June, Barbara and I packed and wrapped fragile items in newspaper, and filled one box after another, loading four truckloads of stuff out of the basement, upstairs and the attic. There were several nice outside toys and a grill from under the stairs leading up to the main house. We gave June what transitional housing could use, and things she could use or she wanted for helping.

A couple of men from church came over to help when service ended. We had my truck loaded down until you couldn't get a piece of newspaper on it, June's truck was packed and the guy had filled his back seat and the trunk of his car full too. We carried three truckloads on my truck and one on June's (although she had a camper shell on hers) over to the church yard, unloading it and covering it up with tarps or plastic until Monday morning.

We had already set out all of the tables and covered them with plastic to keep them from getting wet. We had placed all of our stuff (in totes and boxes) underneath the tables. As we surveyed all of the stuff now sitting in the yard, we knew that we definitely needed to get a very early start the following morning. We didn't have a choice if we expected to get it all set out at a reasonable hour. We stopped at Wendy's on the way home and grabbed something for supper. After working to pack, load, unload and cover all of that stuff we were both too tired to bother with cooking. After eating supper and taking time to grab a quick shower each, we called it an early night.

The following morning was cool and crisp, but with the sun just coming over the horizon, it promised to be another hot day. Sandy had given us a key to the church since we would be there long before she would, just in case we needed to get inside to use the bathroom or wanted to brew a pot of coffee. When we got to the church that morning, we unlocked the church and used the bathroom. Then we held hands in the yard and prayed together. We asked God to bless the sale and all those who would be coming to it before we uncovered the stuff and started working to get it all put out on display

We were shocked at how quickly traffic seemed to start coming by the church as we worked. We had cars pulling into the parking lot, over on the side of the street and even people who were out walking their dogs stopping before we opened the sale. By 8:30, when we had the last item out on the table, Barbara sat down in the chair for a much needed break. She had already sold well over $100 of merchandise and was holding items in reserve that had been paid for and would be picked up later in the day.

Every day that week was the same. We stayed busy and were having to constantly move things on the tables to make room for new items. Several people were bringing donations in boxes and bags and dropping them off behind the chair where we had the cashier's table set up, under one of the biggest trees to allow for shade. By Saturday afternoon when we officially closed the sale, we were absolutely shocked that we had made a total of $950 dollars, and after allowing for gas and food for the week had cleared $850.

The yard sales were not our only accomplishment during this time. We were also blessed in a lot of other ways as well. I was in recovery and although it was going slowly, I felt pretty good compared to a few months earlier. It was hard work, but I was able to load and unload the yard sale equipment and stuff we had for sale on my own. Whenever we held them at the church some of the young men would come and help and I appreciated that. All of the loading and unloading did put a bit of a strain on my shoulder but it wasn't too bad.

The truck we had was a 1987 Chevy S-10 pick up. My mother had helped me buy it from a dealership in Ruckersville back in 1997 so that I would have a way to get back and forth to work when I was working for Capital Interior in Richmond. I had already put two new motors in it and it still had a lot of other small mechanical work that needed to be done to it and at this time we just couldn't afford to spend the money on it. I did basic upkeep and that was about it

It seemed like every day when we checked our mail the majority of it was junk, unless of course you counted bills which never seemed to quit coming. We received one auto sales "gimmick" or another in the mail every week, and we would read it and laugh before ripping it up and throwing it in the trash. Well, we got one from Brown on Route 29. I read and read it and literally worried Barbara to death over it. Well, it caught my attention and I couldn't make my mind up what to do about it.

It sounded like a good deal—$88 a month payment (which of course I knew was just a line to get you into the dealership), but I kept asking her if I should go or if I shouldn't until she got so exasperated she practically ran me out of the house to go. I went and talked to one of the sales associates. He took down all of the information he needed to do an application, except for Barbara's Social Security number. For the life of me I couldn't remember what it was.

As usual, she was on the computer so all I got was a busy signal when I dialed our number. After several tries, I jumped in my truck and went back to the house as fast as I could without getting a speeding ticket. I bounded through the back door of the trailer, about as excited as a starry-eyed child on Christmas morning

"Hurry up! Get off of the computer and call this number and give them your social security number", I yelled, all but shoving the salesman's business card under Barbara's nose. Jerking it out of my hand while laughing at how silly I must have looked, she shut off the computer, and dialed the number. She gave the salesman her social security number and thanked him when he told her that he would call us back when he had some news about our application

We went to church services the next morning, and afterwards, on the drive home we had to go right by the dealership. Barbara suggested that we stop by and ask them if they had heard anything either way on our application. I'm not sure if it was because she thought that we had a chance to be approved, or if she did it so that I wouldn't bug her early the next morning to call them before they had the chance to call us. I wasn't going to debate it and pulled off into the parking lot, finding a spot close to the door so she wouldn't have too far to walk.

I had really liked the young salesman I had spoken with the day before and we waited in the lounge area for him to finish up with a customer he was working with. When he joined us a short time later, he said that because of our income level the only way that he could work out a deal for us was if we had at least $1,000 as a down payment. Well, I thought dejectedly, might as well forget all about this.

He might as well have said we had to have a million and been done with it. There was absolutely no way we could do it. So, totally disappointed, we thanked him and shook his hand and prepared to leave. Barbara said that she had to use the bathroom before we left, so I waited for her to come out before going outside to the truck. When she came out of the bathroom, she walked up to the counter and asked the salesman if we had the $1,000 down payment if we would be able to get a nice used car. It completely shocked me and was so unexpected I couldn't think of a thing to say.

He assured her that we would, but asked her to have a seat while he checked with his manager to be on the safe side. When he rejoined us, Barbara told him that she knew someone who could lend us the money, but that at the moment he was deployed in Iraq; however, he was due to leave for home within the next two weeks. Now it was starting to make sense. She was talking about one of her online friends that she talked to frequently.

He said they were willing to work with that plan if she would be willing to write a post dated check that they could hold until she brought in the money. She agreed but when she reached for her checkbook—Wouldn't you know it? It was the one time that she didn't have even one check left. Damn! Now what were we going to do. Grabbing my keys, I offered to drive back to the house and get a new checkbook. But wait! He said we could bring it in the following day.

I thought we would have to wait until the following day to learn what kind of car we would qualify to get, but he surprised us by saying that he had already picked out the one we could afford the payments on. It was a 2001 Ford Taurus SE Sedan, 4 doors, with tilt-wheel, AC, and many other accessories. And we were going to be able to drive it home that day. Well first we had to finish all of the paperwork and sign it and then allow the shop time to detail the car.

At this point in all of the transactions and talk, I was, shocked, flabbergasted, and dumbfounded—you name it! How had she done it? As the salesman went back to work finalizing the contract, I whispered" how did you come up with that plan? "And she just smiled. Then she said when she had been in the bathroom she had said a prayer: "Lord, you know we need a car, and if it is YOUR will that we have it, show me what to do". I blinked in amazement, and for the first time in a while, was actually speechless.

I knew that it was prayer and God that had brought me through my treatments, my surgery, and recovery and it was clear He was in control of our finances—but a car, too? He really was meeting all of our needs, and I knew it was because we were putting Him front and center in what we were doing

We waited for almost an hour before one of the shop employees pulled the car (silver in color) outside the front door and the salesman walked outside with us to show us all of the features of the car before we left. I liked the style of the car and was surprised the mileage was as low as it read on the odometer.

Barbara, since she was going to be driving it home, got into the driver's seat as the salesman showed her where all of the lights, horn and signals were located, how to adjust the seat (which was electric), and she was paying very close attention to the details. I could tell by the expression on her face she was still in shock, but was also excited and nervous.

This would be the first she had driven since shortly after we'd moved into the trailer park, when we had our Pontiac Grand Am, before the transmission had blown and we had sold it for junk. I'm always giving her pointers on how to drive which she hates, and always tells me to shut up, that she knows how to drive.

She will always follow me on the road or highway because she said when I am behind her it makes her nervous. After being able to get the car I wasn't going to argue with her and I pulled out of the dealership ahead of her. Whenever we got separated, I would pull off to the side of the road and wait for her to catch up again. After a couple of times, it frustrated her and she drove on by me that time, beeping the horn at me. I eventually got ahead of her again, and we pulled into the driveway just a few minutes behind each other. She said that she hadn't had any trouble and that the car drove nice and smooth.

God had definitely blessed us, and that night, as we lay in bed, we gave Him Praise and thanked Him for all which He had done for us and all that He had brought us through. Without Him we wouldn't have been able to do anything and we both knew it.

When Barbara was able to finally get in touch with her friend stationed in Iraq, he was preparing to ship out for the trip back to the States. At that time he didn't have the money to loan her to make the payment at Brown's. We were wondering if we would have to return the car, because the post-dated check was dependant on our being able to take the cash in to replace it. When we called them and explained the situation, we were totally surprised they were willing to work with us to make the payments on the $1,000. For the next three weeks, whenever we held a yard sale, we took a payment to them, and had the amount down to $350.00, and had enough money to buy groceries, pay bills, and even had a little pocket money.

We were still picking up a lot of donations, averaging at least two pick ups per week, so we were busy sorting, cleaning and boxing the items for the next sale. We invested in plastic totes from Family Dollar and Wal-Mart, which were more durable and safer. With the lids they were also much easier to load onto the truck.

We held sales all summer and fall at the church, whenever the weather cooperated. Some weekends we were not able to hold them because it was raining, or was too windy and cold. We had some exciting times that year. Some of the excitement was in a good way and some of it wasn't and came as a total surprise.

Several of the younger guys who were going to the church would help us set out the tables, load heavy items for customers, sell things when it was really busy and oftentimes, help with getting the stuff loaded at the end of the sale, and the yard cleaned for the following week.

We lost a lot of merchandise during one particular sale when a tornado swept through the area, turning tables upside down, blowing stuff through the church yard, and some out into the street. We estimated the loss of items to be well over $300 since some expensive crystal also bit the dust during the calamity. We salvaged a good portion of it and the sale went on.

The following year, the board of directors for the church decided they didn't want any sales held on church property, and we began holding them wherever we could, sometimes having to pay to set them up. It was one reason, besides my recovery, that we opted to stop when we did. None of the other places that we set up really had the high turnover we had enjoyed at the church, although some came close once or twice.

One of the places we set the sale up on a regular basis for a while after leaving the church was at an Antique Shop in Gordonsville. It was closer than the church, only about ten miles from our house. Years before it had been a bar and a dance hall called the "Wooden Nickel." It wasn't as nice as the church and the parking lot itself left a lot to be desired as far as set up and parking arrangements went.

The parking lot had a lot of gravel and some spots were bare, kicking up dust that would cover the stuff we set out for sale and it would get all over the clothing making them appear dirty or stained. It was full of pot holes and often had standing water in a lot of places after a hard rain. There was no shade to speak of and I would often have to take the patio table and umbrella from the deck down there so we would have shade over the cashier's table.

It did have its good points too, though. An elderly gentleman, Carl Ragland, who also lived in Barboursville, operated a produce stand in the parking lot on Fridays, Saturdays and Sundays. He was short, with a low voice, and was always laughing and smiling. He had a very outgoing personality.

He didn't seem to think of anyone as a stranger, and was courteous to all who shopped with him. He always had a great variety of produce and other items for sale, including: tomatoes, cucumbers, cabbage, lettuce, onions and potatoes, bananas, apples, broccoli, zucchini, plums, country ham, fat back, homemade preserves and jellies, apple butter, and seasonal items. Several times he gave us produce that he couldn't keep or that would spoil. We got cucumbers, tomatoes, nectarines, apples, and he was always giving me bunches of banana's. He said the potassium was good for me.

People would stop by to purchase fresh fruits and vegetables from him and out of curiosity, would come over and check out the yard sale at the same time. Sometimes it would be the other way around, where they were drawn to stop because they saw such a big yard sale and would stop to shop with us, and then would also decide to buy from him. It was a very profitable location for both of us.

But it was getting out of hand with all of the stuff we had accumulated, and I was becoming burned out, not having the desire to work them each and every weekend. Barbara had gotten to the point it was hard for her to set the sale up or tear it down without carrying a footstool around to sit on.

We decided to give it up, and gave a good friend of ours a lot of stuff, and donated the rest to people in the area who could use it. We were blessed while it lasted and thanked God for providing for our needs. It was good to have the weekends free again, and my storage shed in the front yard cleared out for my lawn tractor and tools.

A Trip to Remember

In June 2006, at our regular support group meeting, Vikki announced that SPOHNC (pronounced spunk) would be holding their 15th anniversary and Celebration in New York City in mid-August. I listened without giving it much thought as I finished my lunch. After the meeting was over and Vikki, Barbara and I were talking, I made the off-hand comment that it was something I would be very interested in doing if only I had the money to get up there. At the time, I had no idea what that simple statement would set into motion around the hospital.

Vikki began working immediately to figure out a way the cancer center could send Barbara and I to New York, with all expenses paid. It wasn't only because I had said I wanted to go, but Second Wind, being a charter member of SPOHNC, would have representation at the event. Before Vikki said anything to us about it, she contacted the staff of the cancer center, a student organization who donated toward worthy causes of the center, John Conover, and the Hope Fund.

All of the contacts she made and all of the planning was done to find money to pay for transportation, the registration fee for the conference itself, and of course the cost of the hotel room. When she had the funds, she called and told us we would be able to go to New York. Barbara and I were both shocked and very excited. We could hardly believe that Vikki had worked so hard to put together the money because I had said that I was interested in going. I knew that she wanted our group to be represented and recognized, but it was still a shock that she had done it.

It would be the first time I had traveled to New York, and although Barbara had traveled some to other states (Florida, Pennsylvania, West Virginia, North Carolina, Georgia, South Carolina and Washington, DC) before we were married, I had not. I had lived in Richmond and for a brief time in Danville, and all around the local area. But I hadn't really done any travel to speak of outside the state of Virginia.

Vikki said she had arranged it so we would be riding Amtrak—(my first train ride too! This was getting better all the time), and that our hotel and registration would also be included. It would be up to us to raise money for incidentals or emergency use while we were gone, and she suggested that we come up with at least $100 in pocket money to tide us over. All of this happened before we had stopped holding the weekly yard sales, so we were pretty sure that we would have no problem in saving back the money.

We were both excited, and had something to look forward to that we would enjoy together. We began thinking ahead to the outfits we would pack for the event, wondering if it would be casual or business type clothing that would be required. To be sure, Barbara telephone Janine Cortese, the Office Manager of SPOHNC to find out. It was business casual so we didn't really need to take anything fancy. We also debated whether or not we should take Barbara's manual wheelchair. It would definitely make mobility easier for Barbara instead of trying to walk and aggravate her back, but at the same time it would definitely be a hassle worrying about it being put on and taken off of the train. In the end we decided to leave it at home, and use ones available at the train station. We could check once we got there to see if they had one at the hotel that she could use if she needed to.

A couple days before we were to leave, Vikki called and said there was a glitch that needed to be ironed out. Unfortunately, the Amtrak ride was out, because when she called to confirm our reservation for two seats, she discovered a problem. On the day we were to arrive in New York, there wasn't a train that could get us there at the time we needed. She said she would call us back when she had the details worked out.

We were left dangling in suspense for a little over a day. We waited anxiously to hear back from her on how we would be traveling. We had the money we had saved, and Barbara had packed our bags with appropriate clothing, toiletries and accessories (including a lot of film for pictures if the opportunity arose) that we would need while there. Finally, the day before the trip, we got the call.

We would be flying round trip on United from the Charlottesville-Albemarle Airport into LaGuardia Airport in New York. WHOAH!! Did you say fly? Me—get on an airplane—way up there? I wasn't too sure about that one; I'd never been in any kind of transportation where my feet weren't planted on solid ground, unless you counted the carnival rides at a fair. Barbara, mouth hanging open in surprise, said uh ho, no way. If God wanted me to fly, then He'd have given me wings! Of course, we had this entire conversation once we weren't on the phone with Vikki. We didn't want to disappoint her after all of the hard work she had put into the project. We also didn't want to do anything to jeopardize our going. What the hell, I thought. Flying can't be that bad can it? I mean people do it everyday.

Vikki told us that since the cancer center was paying for the transportation and other expenses, she would make it easier for us and would drive out to the airport and pay for the tickets. She would leave them at the ticket counter for us, and when we got there all we would need was our driver's licenses to pick up our boarding passes for the plane

We weren't sure how our bodies would react to flying so to be on the safe side; the morning of our flight we left the house a little early. We wanted to allow enough time to stop by the store to pick up some Dramamine Tablets for motion sickness just in case we needed them. Barbara had filled all of our prescriptions and had made sure she picked up enough cigarettes to last for the trip because we knew they were probably expensive in New York.

Traffic was fairly light on the road as we drove into Charlottesville. When we arrived at the airport, I pulled up to the front entrance and went to find a wheelchair for Barbara. I pushed her into the lobby where it was cool, while I went to park the car in the designated parking lot. Our luggage was the kind that had wheels built into the base with a handle to pull them, so I decided to park before unloading them from the trunk. When I rejoined Barbara inside the lobby, we proceeded to the ticket counter like Vikki had told us to, and we each had our driver's licenses in our hand. Did we ever receive one hell of a shock when we gave our names?

When the ticket agent, (a middle-aged man who looked frazzled from dealing with the number of people demanding his attention), typed in our names, he said the computer showed we were supposed to come back from New York on Sunday afternoon (which was right), and in the next breath, he said he couldn't find our tickets any where in his computer system.

Excuse me? What did he mean, we weren't in the system? How could we be coming back to a place that we hadn't left? We asked him to check again and he did. He double checked every thing two or three times, and kept coming up with the same results. He finally called the cancer center, and then had Vikki paged through the operator, and didn't get an answer. He finally threw his hands up in the air in total defeat. The line behind us was getting longer and longer and he was getting more frazzled with each passing second.

He started writing out two boarding passes by hand. Handing them over at last, he cautioned us to be sure to keep them in a safe place, because no more could be issued if we lost them. We thanked him, and pulling our luggage, went to find a restroom. Then we wanted to get something cold to drink since we had a while before we had to board the plane.

After using the restroom and freshening up, we went outside so Barbara could smoke and to finish our cold drinks. We thought this would be a good time to take the Dramamine so it would have time to work before the plane took off. We sat outside for several minutes, finishing our drinks while Barbara enjoyed smoking a cigarette, and we watched all of the different people coming into the airport. Some chose to come in taxis, while others had family and friends drop them off, and others opted to use the parking lot and pay when they returned.

We had been warned about how tight the airport security checks would be, so we headed back inside to get through all of the formality. The terrorist attacks of September 11, 2001 had changed our lives here in the United States forever. There were always news reports of the alert system bouncing back and forth so much it made a person dizzy; airport security was tightened to the point it took passengers forever to be screened and checked in.

The list of items you could no longer carry on a flight seemed to grow daily. We were aware of what was and wasn't allowed, and had packed accordingly. All of our liquids (including my Ensure) which I had a letter from Dr. Read that would allow me to consume them on the flight, were in our check-in baggage.

We were walked through a scanner, similar to that in a Federal Courthouse, with our bags on the conveyor belt along with Barbara's purse. The baggage and purse were examined inside and out, and then we were frisked and patted down—my wife by a lady security guard, myself by a man.

Finally, after several minutes, we were free to go to the lounge area, where we could watch planes landing and taking off. They had told us that Barbara would be taken out to the plane in the wheelchair by a woman security guard, who would help her board the plane.

Our seats on the boarding pass were located in the front section of the plane. As we stepped aboard, the stewardess asked us if we would move further back. We each took window seats across the aisle from each other. The windows were overlooking, of all things, the wings. I curiously looked around the inside of the plane. The ones you see in movies are so big and spacious with a lot of head and leg room. I wondered what kind of plane they used to shoot those scenes. It wasn't a plane like we found ourselves sitting in right now.

The seats were close together, one behind the other, and Barbara, being on the heavy side—(she hates when I mention her weight) had problems finding a comfortable position in which she wasn't cramped.

Not only were her legs cramped up and she couldn't stretch them out, but the seat didn't recline enough for her to find a comfortable position to take the pressure off of her lower back and right hip. The plane was quite small on the inside; nothing like it looked to be from the ground. The bathroom, located at the back of the plane would prove toward the end of the flight to be something that definitely left a lot to be desired.

It was hot and very muggy inside the plane because the air conditioning wouldn't begin to work until after take off and we were actually in flight. I noticed that the heat and humidity must be affecting her breathing, because Barbara dug her inhaler out of her purse and took two puffs of it as we were waiting for final instructions from the pilot.

Take-off wasn't as bad as I had imagined that it would be, although my stomach did a little dip, but it was nothing major. I watched out of the window as the ground slowly fell away, becoming little more than a speck far, far below as we picked up altitude and speed after being cleared by the tower. I glanced over at Barbara to give her an encouraging smile, but found that she was busy watching out of the window. We flew over the trailer park where we live! Way cool, I thought. Hey you guys look up. I'm up here, flying over top of you this morning!

Food! I need food I thought, as my stomach began growling not too long after we were in the air. We'd been in a hurry when we left home, and not wanting to get sick, neither of us had done more than have a couple cups of coffee. Now my body began protesting quite loudly.

The stewardess must have read my mind, because she brought out the—Holy cow! You've got to be kidding, I groaned. Flat ginger ale, tepid at best, and chips that definitely tasted well past the freshness date on the package. The chips were almost impossible for me to chew, because I'd had all of my teeth extracted, but my gums had not healed enough to get dentures.

I had to eat easily digested, soft food, and neither of these fit the bill. I managed to finish them by allowing them to soften in my mouth before trying to chew them, then washing them down with the ginger ale. Well, at least it was wet.

Halfway through the flight, my bladder alerted me it was time to use the little boy's room. I unbuckled my seat belt, stepped into the aisle and walked toward the end of the plane where it was located. As I stepped inside, with barely enough room to stand to comfortably do business, the heat from the engines of the plane made it stifling. I finished as quickly as possible, taking a deep breath when I came back into the body of the plane.

I made my way back to my seat. Thankfully, it was cooler out here. A short time later, Barbara (and I know she was hoping she could wait until New York) had to get up to go to the bathroom. I saw her hesitate before opening the door and stepping in.

The door didn't want to stay closed, and in just a few minutes, she literally burst back into the plane, gasping for air. I know it had been hard for her to breathe inside, and perspiration was beaded on her face, which she swiped off with the back of her hand as she sat down and reconnected the seat belt. She shook her head at me, and rolled her eyes, as if to say "UNBELIEVABLE!"

The flight went smoothly and was relatively uneventful. I was excited as we began our dissent and approach into New York and LaGuardia. Then I heard my wife gasp out loud as the plane hit a large pocket of air turbulence, rocking back and forth several times until it settled back down.

The pilot hastened to assure us everything was fine and that it was just a pocket of unstable air. I was watching out of the window as we flew over Ground Zero. It was hard to believe that tiny little spot on the ground far below had been the site of one of the worse tragedies to happen on US soil in the history of our country. I also got to see an aerial view of the East River, and downtown Manhattan in the distance, and Shea Stadium as we approached the airport. We also saw the Statue of Liberty in the distance. That was one thing that I had always wanted to do, visit it and climb to the top. Well, one of these days I thought, as I felt the plane begin to drop altitude and prepare for it's landing, which I prayed went smoothly.

The stewardess had assured us she that she had radioed ahead to the ground crew at LaGuardia that we needed a wheelchair on standby. They had responded, confirming one would be waiting. Once the doors were opened, we were asked to wait because the wheelchair was not there yet.

It was hot and stifling on the plane, and we were forced to wait for about forty-five minutes before an employee finally came out with one. Barbara's legs and back had gotten stiff from sitting during the flight and it took her several minutes to navigate the steep steps of the airplane to the ground below. She gratefully sank down into the wheelchair at the bottom of the steps.

We both exhaled sighs of relief as the coolness of the air conditioning washed over us like a soothing balm when we entered the sliding doors of the airport. The employee pushing the wheelchair took us to the baggage claim area where we had to wait in line for our luggage.

The next stop was to find a real restroom, where we could wash our faces and get a cool drink. It was a relief for both of us to walk into a normal size bathroom and not feel like we were going to be stifled as we used the facility. After joining back up, the first thing that we needed to concentrate on was getting to the LaGuardia Marriott where we would be staying.

I couldn't believe the size of this airport! In contrast to the one in Charlottesville, LaGuardia was absolutely amazing. It seemed to stretch for miles and miles, with services located everywhere you looked. There were ATM's, shoe shine stands, Taxi stands, newspapers and magazines, ice cream Shoppe's, fast food restaurants, the list went on and on.

We had received a letter from SPOHNC before the trip that confirmed our reservations for the conference and celebration, and in it had been instructions on how to summon the shuttle bus to the hotel. It was a free service they offered to all of their guests. We were supposed to find the LaGuardia Marriott hotel phone, and when we lifted the receiver, it would ring at the hotel. They would then send their shuttle over to pick us up and bring us to the main entrance. That sounded simple enough and should be easy.

We had a major problem: not only did we not see the telephone, but there was a language barrier. Barbara and I tried unsuccessfully over and over again to make the airport employees (most who were Spanish and not good at English) understand what it was that we were looking for. Even after reading the letter we showed to them, they were dumbfounded, and ended up shrugging their shoulders, at a complete loss how to help us.

Finally, after we had almost become so frustrated we could have screamed, we found a young lady who worked at the airport who understood exactly what we were looking for. We were more than a little embarrassed to discover that we had been standing within a few feet of the damn telephone the whole time. I went over and picked up the receiver waiting for the hotel to answer. When they did, I gave my name and location at the airport and they said that the shuttle would be over to pick us up within a few minutes.

We made our way through the crowd (who were all hustling and bustling to get where they were going, rushing along as if they were racing to a fire, oblivious of those around them), to the front of the airport to wait for the shuttle.

Almost immediately, Barbara dug out her cigarettes and matches (still smarting at the fact that security in Charlottesville had confiscated her brand new lighter) and lit one, inhaling a deep drag from it and relishing the taste before exhaling.

Watching the taxi drivers constantly zipping in and out of the traffic there in front of the airport was absolutely amazing. And I thought that people in Virginia were bad drivers and acted stupid! They would pull right out in front of each other, horns honking repeatedly, or would zip out right in front of the big buses, coming within mere inches of being hit or run over. How they avoided major collisions was anybody's guess.

We weren't used to things at such a fast pace. We were both reading all of the shuttle buses signs as they drove up, and were worried that we would miss the one the hotel was sending over. After waiting for what seemed like hours, I went back into the airport to try calling the hotel again. Wouldn't you know it? As soon as I did, the damn shuttle showed up and I had to rush to make it back in time to get on board. The road to the hotel went over several bridges that were in sad need of repair, jostling the bus so much it made you raise up and down on the seat like you were a jack in the box. Barbara finally complained to me that it made her teeth actually rattle, and it was giving her a headache. I wondered if the headache wasn't coming from the fact that neither of us had eaten very much all day, and it was approaching late afternoon.

It had definitely been quite an experience getting to New York, and I was feeling very fatigued by now. All I knew was that we were both looking forward to stretching out on the bed in our room and cooling off in the air conditioning. It would also definitely be nice to have something to snack on. I was beginning to feel very nauseated from not eating much. It was probably why I was feeling so tired and weak too.

As we entered the hotel through the automatic double doors, I was very impressed. There were crystal chandelier lights trimmed in gold hanging from the ceiling, and the tile floors gleamed as if someone had spent hours buffing and waxing them. There was a formal sitting area off to the left of the entrance that had been arranged in a formal living room style, with deep burgundy and striped sofas, with paisley print wing chairs arranged at an angle, and the tables were a deep dark cherry wood that gleamed and sparkled with the light reflecting off of them. The carpet on that part of the floor looked to be so thick your feet would sink down when you walked on it. There were beautiful silk plants arranged through the sitting area and down the hallway, some in gold planters and some in pewter style ones.

The registration desk stood to the right of the entrance and took up almost half of the area. It stood just at chest level and was a deep dark mahogany. Behind the counter stood the Assistant Manager of the hotel, who welcomed us warmly as we approached him. We gave our names and he typed them into the computer system.

He told us that we were indeed registered to attend the conference and celebration and then floored us by asking how we would like to pay for our room. Which credit card we would prefer to use? My mouth fell open and I was so shocked that for several seconds I couldn't utter a sound. What did he mean, pay for the room? There had to be some mistake!

Barbara and I both explained to him that Vikki Bravo from the cancer center at the University of Virginia had made all of the arrangements and that the room had already been paid for. He told us that the only thing his records showed as having been paid was the registration fee charged by SPOHNC for the event. Damn! Here we were miles from home, and we didn't have a room? Good Lord! What were we going to do now? Barbara just laid her head down on the counter of the desk.

With effort she pulled herself together and gave him the telephone number of the page operator at the hospital, and he called, trying to page Vikki but got no response. She was probably in a meeting of some sort and couldn't answer the page. We were dumbfounded and at a complete loss on what to do about the situation. We certainly didn't have the money to pay for the room and our flight home wasn't until Sunday, two days away. He briefly excused himself and walked off down one of the hallways.

I asked Barbara what the hell could have happened since all of this was supposed to have been taken care of before we left home, and she didn't know any more than I did. We stood at the registration desk, worried and tired, and not knowing what would happen when the Assistant Manager came back. Well, I thought—this is one hell of a mess. No room, I'm tired, and I'm hungry. Part of me was beginning to wish I had never opened my mouth at that support group when Vikki first mentioned this event.

After we had waited for several long and agonizing minutes we saw him coming back up the hall and with him was a short petite woman wearing a nice business suit. Well, he has gone and found the Manager; I remember thinking to myself as I saw them approach the desk. When he continued to walk behind the desk while the woman approached us, I was confused.

That confusion turned to utter embarrassment within thirty seconds after she introduced herself as the President and Founder of SPOHNC! He had gone in search of Nancy Leupold! Oh my God! This is definitely not good, I thought. It certainly isn't how I envisioned meeting the president of the nationally recognized organization that our little group was a member of. What must she think?

Barbara and I each shook her hand as she introduced herself, and quickly apologized for having to bother her with our predicament. She brushed it aside with a wave of her hand, saying that she was certain it was just some small mix-up. She turned to the Assistant Manager who was waiting patiently behind the desk and, handing him a credit card, asked him to charge our room to the organization. She told him that a room should be available because she had received a call from someone who had been unable to make it to the event at the last moment.

Nancy smiled and shook our hands again, telling us to enjoy the event and made her way back down the hall to resume whatever she had been working on before being interrupted. The Assistant Manager gave us the keys to our room which he told us was located on the second floor, and we walked to the elevator. Neither of us said a word as it zipped us upward to what I could only hope would be a nice room.

New Places, New Faces

When we unlocked our room with the card and stepped inside, we were quite surprised. It was beautifully decorated and spacious. The furniture was dark cherry and was polished to a glowing shine, well taken care of, and arranged to be comfortable but not crowded.

There was a huge king-size bed with a heavy white quilted spread and decorative sham pillows, with summer prints hanging above the cherry headboard, and one on the short wall toward the bathroom. The furniture consisted of a cherry armoire that housed the television and VCR at the top, while the middle was a "bar", complete with ice bucket and a place to set drinks, etc. The doors would slide closed when the television or bar wasn't in use. Underneath were several drawers for storage.

The large cherry dresser had a total of eight drawers, four on each side and a large mirror attached at the top. Beside it, close to the window was a writing table/desk, with a gleaming gold table lamp and crisp white shade, and the telephone. It was also set up for wireless internet service for those who had brought their laptop computers with them. If Barbara had thought about it she probably would have packed her laptop, but I guess she figured she wouldn't have time to use it anyway.

The window, with its vertical blinds, opened to reveal just a parking lot which wasn't very interesting, although we did get to watch several beautiful sunsets while we were there. It was awesome to watch it going down over the NYC skyline, with the sky-scrapers and other buildings on the horizon.

They had also provided a place to "kick back" if writing or computer and the other amenities didn't appeal to you and you weren't ready for bed. There was a very comfortable Queen Anne style wing chair and ottoman positioned in the corner, between the bed and the window. The closet space was just inside the room door, across from the bathroom, and had built in hangers on steel rods with shelf space for luggage on top and open space on the floor at the bottom.

Barbara and I were both tired, and all I wanted to do was to kick off my shoes and stretch out on the bed for a nap. Right then I didn't care if it was made out of concrete and mortar. I just needed to lie down before I collapsed and fell flat on my face. I was pleasantly surprised to discover that it was very comfortable, but the pillows weren't very good. They were more like toss pillows that you would use on a sofa or loveseat and not a bed. It didn't take very long and I was napping quite contentedly.

As I napped, Barbara went downstairs and outside to the smoking area to have a cigarette and relax for a few minutes. When she returned to the room, she took her time and unpacked all of our clothes, shaking them out before hanging them up. We had packed them carefully, and most of them were Permanent Press. She put all of our toiletry items in the bathroom and then took a cool sponge bath before joining me on the bed for a nap herself.

A short time later my stomach woke me up by rumbling non-stop, reminding me that I hadn't fed it properly all day. I decided that it was definitely time to go rustle up some food. The confirmation letter had told us that we needed to buy our dinner for tonight. Most of the people who were going to attend the event weren't expected to arrive until later tonight or early on Saturday morning.

When we had entered the hotel I had been looking at the lobby and how it was set up, and then with the mix up about the room it hadn't occurred to me to find out about what restaurants were located in the hotel, or perhaps within easy walking distance. After washing our face and brushing our teeth and hair to look presentable we left the room and went in search of dinner.

We took the elevator back to the lobby and asked about restaurants at the registration desk. There were actually two eating establishments inside the hotel, down the hallway past the elevators. The first one was a formal one, where people got "dressed" for dinner which we didn't feel we should try. We were dressed nice but not formal and we would have stuck out like a sore thumb, so we walked on by it to the second one.

This one was more our style and to our liking. It was designed like a "pub" or sports bar. There were several televisions mounted on the walls in different areas and they each had a different ball game in progress. It was fairly busy, but not crowded. There was a long mahogany bar in the center of the room with padded leather bar stools down the entire length, and then there were smaller tables set at different angles around the room. There were also booths located along the back wall, which is where we decided to sit. The tables weren't bolted to the floor which meant neither of us would be cramped, and we could stretch out our legs and relax.

The waitress came over a few minutes after we'd taken our seats and handed each of us a menu, asking what we would like to drink. Opening the menu, my eyes nearly bulged out of my head when I saw the price list. I understood now why Vikki had insisted we bring extra spending money! My God, at these prices it was a good thing the rest of the food and refreshments would be provided by the hotel as part of the event, or we would have starved to death or died of thirst by the time we got back home.

Barbara's favorite foods had always chicken and beef in that order and she said she was definitely looking forward to enjoying a nice thick, juicy hamburger with lettuce, tomato, mayonnaise and onions and a basket of French fries to go with it. Well, it wasn't going to happen if we had to order it here. The closest thing they had on the menu to a regular hamburger was called a "Shea Burger "(evidently because you could see Shea Stadium from the front of the hotel), and the damn thing was $13.95!

We went through the menu together and finally decided to order a deluxe pizza with everything except anchovies and olives to share. I ordered a Budweiser in the bottle and she ordered a large Pepsi. After we placed our order and were waiting for the food to arrive, Barbara went out to the lobby where she had noticed the registration tables set up by SPOHNC.

We were required to register for the Continental Breakfast and the start of the Conference the next morning. She picked up the information packets which also included our name tags, that they asked us to wear at all times whenever we were out of our room.

Barbara had spoken with Janine Cortese, the Office Manager of SPOHNC several times on the telephone before our trip, and it was finally nice for her to be able to put a face with the voice. Janine was working the table, and was distributing the registration packets. She was tall and slender, with red hair cut in an attractive page style, and was very outgoing and friendly. Barbara chatted with her for several minutes after receiving the packet.

Nancy eventually joined the conversation when she came out of one of the Salons after checking on the preparations for the conference the following morning. The ENT Clinic had been gracious enough to provide us with several VCR and CD Rom presentations of Larry's exercise program we could leave with Nancy for her collection

After talking with them, Barbara rejoined me in the restaurant, and we at our dinner slowly, savoring the taste and just spending the time finally relaxing after a very long and trying day. We had been rushing around non-stop ever since we got out of bed that morning. We'd showered, gulped down a couple cups of coffee each, stopping to buy the Dramamine and rushing to the airport for the flight. By now I just felt like I didn't want to move any more than I had to and wanted to chill out before bedtime. We talked about small things: the flight, the attitude of the people at the airport, any and everything that was light and didn't really require thinking or planning. When the waitress brought the tab for the meal the total (we'd each gotten refills on our drinks) was $26.95. Wow! I was really glad this was the only meal we had to buy during the trip. After paying the bill, we decided that we would go out to the smoking area in front of the hotel for a while and just enjoy being in New York.

We sat down on one of two wide slotted wooden benches, made from oak that was well seasoned, and were set on each side of the main entrance. I looked around the area, surprised at how well kept and maintained it was. There were iron planters that held petunias, daffodils and multi-colored blooms all around the area, with a high white masonry wall that overlooked the highway below. The area was well-lit, with huge square lights in the roof over the sitting area, and entrance, as well as lights on cement posts located in the median that separated the circular drive from the parking area around to the hotel entrance.

Tonight, there was a rather gusty breeze, humid but not stifling, as we settled back to relax. The night was clear and there were a million stars shining in the midnight blue sky overhead. The high wall on one side shielded the noise of the traffic below until it was like muted surf, with horns sounding far off and not right outside of the wall.

As we sat there in silence, we watched as people came and went and there were several large groups that we assumed were some of the people who would be at the conference for the weekend. More than a few smiled and said hello as they passed us, all very friendly. There were several young men in fatigues milling around in a group, laughing and talking among themselves, who spoke to us as we sat down. One of them noticed the name tags we had on, and asked about the celebration.

The conversation skipped from one subject to the other—and we discovered that they were all members of a National Guard Troop from Kentucky, who had just come home after a tour of duty in Iraq, and were now staying at the hotel when not on guard duty over at LaGuardia.

Barbara and I had written lots of letters to our troops stationed overseas—especially in Iraq, as part of our church's outreach ministry, and it was a pleasure to meet them in person—to thank them for their sacrifices in defending our country and to welcome them home.

We both had a lot of questions about what it had been like over in that country while they were stationed there, but thinking that it was a subject that they didn't want to talk about, we were hesitant to ask the questions. A couple of them did tell about how sandy it was, and how they had to learn how to deal with all of the heat and other inconveniences of being in a war zone constantly. They all talked about how friendly and desperate the children were to make friends, and that most of the people welcomed the presence of our military over there to help them. Over the course of our stay, we were able to have several conversations with them, and it was one of the highlights of the trip for both of us.

We went back up to our room a little while later, both of us exhausted since the day had finally caught up with us both. I felt like I just couldn't hold my head up another minute. I stripped off my clothes and all but collapsed on the mattress pulling the heavy spread over top of me and plumping the pillows to try and get them more comfortable under my head. Barbara undressed and took a long hot shower before calling the front desk and asking for a wake-up call at six the following morning so we wouldn't be late for breakfast before crawling in bed and falling asleep almost as soon as her head touched the pillow.

THE EXPERTS SPEAK

The insistent ringing of the telephone roused me from a deep slumber at six O'clock the next morning. With fumbling fingers, I drowsily searched for it, lifting it up and bringing it to my ear, roughly saying" hello", only to hear a recording say it was our requested wake up call. I dropped the receiver none too gently back onto the base and rolled over.

I reached over gently shaking Barbara's shoulder, telling her it was time to get up. I was very surprised that she hadn't heard the telephone ringing. Moving over and snuggling against me with her head on my shoulder, she asked how I'd slept. "Like a baby", I said, laughing. Surprisingly, I had, considering it was a strange bed. Once I fell asleep I didn't move the whole night and never even got up to use the bathroom. Man, I must have been wiped out I thought; I usually get up and down all through the night at home to go to the bathroom.

After lying there for several minutes, I got up and headed for the shower while Barbara got our clothes out we would wear for the day. She came into the bathroom to make a pot of coffee in the 2-cup coffeemaker supplied by the hotel. Since she had taken a shower the night before, she brushed her teeth and applied her make up and earrings and then got dressed and was ready by the time I got out of the shower to towel off.

We knew that the maid service of the hotel would tidy the room and make the bed, so while I was getting dressed Barbara left the room with her cup of coffee to go to the smoking area downstairs. I told her that I would meet her downstairs in a little while so we could go to breakfast. I was really looking forward to it. The pizza and beer from dinner were gone and my stomach wanted food.

We had read over some of the information included in the packet Barbara picked up during registration, and learned it had taken two years to plan and organize the celebration and conference. The list of guest speakers and the topics that would be covered in the two-day event were amazing.

The panel of guests were from all across the United States and the topics that were being included were on subjects of interest and importance to all cancer patients, survivors and caregivers as well as family members. I knew that Barbara had been certain to pack a generous supply of steno and legal pads and pens so that she could take lots of notes for our group and for our own personal use.

When I finished getting dressed I made myself a cup of coffee, and after turning off the coffeemaker, I met Barbara outside in the smoking area. We sat on the bench to finish our coffee, enjoying the cool morning breeze that was blowing. We knew that it would probably get hot and muggy before the day was over, but for now it was very comfortable. We made our way inside to enjoy the Continental Breakfast provided by the hotel. The menu looked good and my stomach growled appreciatively as I stood in line. Barbara had gone to find us a seat at one of the tables since the line was long and growing by the minute. It would have caused her back to feel like it was falling in half to stand for that long.

There was so much to choose from it was hard to decide what to put on our plates. There was a variety of Danish Muffins, Breakfast Breads, Croissants and Assorted Bagels, Assorted Cream Cheeses, Butter, Margarine, Preserves and Honey, Sliced Seasonal Fruit, Assorted Flavored Yogurts and Individual Kellogg's Cereals, Orange, Cranberry and Grapefruit Juices, Bottled Water, Freshly Brewed Gourmet Bean 100% Arabica Blend, Premium Roast Coffee, Brewed Decaffeinated Coffee and International Assorted Teas. I chose a bagel and some fruit and a croissant for Barbara along with coffee and juice and then went back and got myself cereal, some fresh seasonal fruit, a muffin and orange juice and coffee.

As the wait staff of the hotel began clearing away the food, the conference began. Up in the front of the room there was a long table set up for the guest speakers. Nancy Leupold welcomed everyone who came, outlined the events of the conference, talked about the founding of SPOHNC and how much it has grown over the years.

The first speaker following Nancy's speech was Dr. William Ravich, M.D., who is the Clinical Director of the Swallowing Center at Johns Hopkins Medicine.

His presentation was on the different techniques and new swallowing therapies which had been developed to help head and neck cancer patients overcome problems with eating and drinking during and after treatment.

He was followed by Dorothy Villano and Diane Saulie—both from North Shore LIJ Health Care Systems, who added more aspects of the same topic. Barbara was listening attentively, and her pen never seemed to leave the paper as she quickly flipped pages and filled them at an astounding rate, never losing concentration.

At 10:00 a.m., we took a break for refreshments and to visit with the different Vendors who had set up Exhibits of materials ranging from samples of lozenges for dry mouth, coupons for savings, cookbooks, bracelets and necklaces offered by SPOHNC, survivorship notebooks offered by the Lance Armstrong Foundation, the list went on and on. I watched as Barbara began making her way through the vendors, gathering stack after stack, and finding ones that offered tote bags which she filled to overflowing.

She took them back into the main room, sitting them down and then going outside with her soda to have a cigarette before returning for the next presentation.

The next presentation was on Acupuncture Treatment for Dry Mouth in Head and Neck Cancer Patients and was presented by Richard C. Niemtzow, M.D., Director of the Acupuncture Clinic at Andrews Air Force Base, MD.

His presentation yielded about four pages of notes and lasted for forty minutes. I was starting to feel really tired—probably jet lag, and returned to the room to rest before we were supposed to meet for a buffet lunch. I took the materials Barbara had already gathered with me when I went to the room.

I knew that she had promised Vikki that she would take notes and bring back a lot of information for the group, so I knew that she would be staying for a while longer at the conference. I stepped outside for a few minutes of air and made my way to the room.

The presentation before lunch was on Mind/Body Medicine: Keys to Survivorship for Cancer Patients and was given by Ann Webster, PhD, Director of Mind/Body programs for cancer at Harvard Medical

School. It was one of the presentations where Barbara did not take notes—only one of two that she didn't attend.

When she joined me a little while later, she said that the presentation before lunch wasn't very interesting, and the carpal tunnel syndrome in her right hand was flaring up. She said she needed to rest it before the afternoon session started. She kicked off her shoes and joined me on the bed for a quick power nap before we went down for lunch, being held in the Liberty Suite on the Lobby Level.

When we walked in, we couldn't believe the amount of food and the selection! There were cold salads and soups including: Caesar Salad, Romaine with Caesar Dressing and Grated Parmesan Cheese, Roasted Garlic Croutons, Portobello and Artichoke Salad, Italian Bread and Olive Oil, Chilled Vichyssoise. Then there was a great selection of Hot Entrees including: Roasted Basil crusted Chicken served with Vegetable Risotto with Tomato Confit, Jumbo Ricotta Cheese Ravioli on Fresh Zucchini and Topped with Wilted Baby Spinach, Assorted Rolls and Butter. As with the Continental breakfast that morning, there was a variety of beverages, included bottled water, coffee, tea and diet and regular sodas.

Barbara and I both went to the presentation after lunch. It was about advances in Treatment for Head and Neck Cancer that was given by David I. Rosenthal, M.D., and Director of Head and Neck Translational Research Department of Radiation Oncology at M.D. Anderson Cancer Center; Marshall Posner, M.D., Director of Head and Neck Oncology Program, Dana-Farber Cancer Institute and Adam S. Jacobson, MD, from the Department of Otolaryngology Mt. Sinai Medical Center, NY.

Vikki had worked at M.D. Anderson Cancer Center before she transferred to the University of Virginia, and when we mentioned her to Dr. Rosenthal that night, his face lit up. He said that he remembered her quite well and for us to tell her hello from him when we returned home. He casually asked me questions about my treatments and how things were going, and he seemed genuinely interested in what I had to say.

I also met another guy who was just starting out in his treatments and as he talked about them, I realized that he had been diagnosed with the same cancer I had and that his treatments would mirror the ones I had gone through. I can't remember his name or where he was from, but what he said really impressed me and stuck in my memory. He had the attitude that he would abide by what his healthcare team suggested as far as the treatment plan went, but when it came to suggesting that he apply for disability and not work, he was not listening. The cancer had invaded his body, but it wasn't going to control his ability to live like he always had. I wonder how long he was able to stand by his guns, or if somewhere along the line, he changed his mind?

The one presentation that Vikki had specifically asked Barbara to attend and take notes on was the last one of the day: Medically Necessary Dental Care, given by Sally Hart, Esquire, and an attorney with the Arizona Center for Disability Law, In Tucson, and Consulting Counsel for Center for Medicare Advocacy in Connecticut. There were a lot of patients being diagnosed at the University who were having problems not only with the oral hygiene, but were dealing with Medicare's attitude about providing coverage for it.

Maybe it was because I was tired, or bored, or maybe even feeling a little neglected, who knows. Hell, maybe it was even a combination of all three. Barbara and I got into an argument when she got ready to leave the room for the meeting while I was lying down on the bed. I felt like a heel when she left the room with tears in her eyes, carrying her notepads. As I drifted off for a nap, I knew I'd have to find a way to make it up to her later. We both apologized to each other for losing our temper. I really was sorry for the way I acted because the main reason that we had come to the event was to find out information that could help me and all of the other cancer patients, and she couldn't do that if she had stayed cooped up in the hotel room with me because I didn't want to go to the meetings.

I was really looking forward to the meal on this, our last night in New York. It was a reception that was being held in the Grand Ballroom of the hotel. It was in honor of the founding of SPOHNC and from the menu listed in our information packet it sounded liked the food would be delicious too.

The reception was scheduled to start at 6:30 so Barbara and I rushed from the last presentation to the room to be able to take a shower and get dressed. We had tote bags full of samples, notebooks, water bottles and other stuff we had collected and we just added them to the previous ones on the floor beside the desk.

When we arrived downstairs and entered the banquet, it was breathtaking. All of the tables were beautifully set and decorated; with lighted candles, starched white tablecloths and napkins, that when combined with the dimmed lighting in the room gave it a relaxed and intimate atmosphere. We found a table near the entrance and joined a festive group who looked ready to relax, and enjoy good food and each other's company for the evening. Barbara and I were both shocked to discover that they were serving both bottled beer and wine with the menu. This was definitely my style I thought as I headed for the bar area and a cold beer, bringing Barbara back a glass of white wine that she barely touched the whole evening. She decided to drink Pepsi and eventually got a nice cold fruit punch.

I spent the time eating and enjoying the food, and chatting with Dr. Rosenthal who was seated beside me to my right, and a survivor from out in the Midwest beside Barbara. The food Barbara and I found that we liked the best was the Pasta and Potato stations, Beef Tenderloin and the raw vegetables. I couldn't eat those so I went for the beef and the Maryland Crab cakes. I was still sipping on a beer when she was ready to leave and I told her to go ahead and I would meet her outside later.

As we were relaxing out front later, a black limousine pulled up to the front, and we did a double take at first when one of the porters came through the front door, pushing one of the luggage carriers, and sitting on it in a chair was Little Richard!

Barbara had her purse with her, and was frantically trying to find her camera that she kept with her to snap a picture of him. With all of the medication and other necessities she had in it, by the time she got it out, not only had his luggage been loaded but he was in the limousine and it was pulling away from the hotel. She was totally disappointed, vowing she was definitely going to clean out her purse as soon as we got back home.

TEARS AND LAUGHTER

Early Sunday morning, after once again receiving a wake up call from the front desk, we got out of bed and started a pot of coffee brewing while we began packing for the trip home. Nancy had made the announcement yesterday during the conference that the hotel had generously extended the check out time for the guests attending the conference until one O'clock in the afternoon, after the conclusion of the conference.

Barbara and I wanted to be ready to leave immediately afterwards, and didn't want to feel like we were being rushed out of the place, and take a chance that we would forget and leave something behind. We had a lot to repack and because our flight home was scheduled to take off at three O'clock, we needed to be at LaGuardia no later than two O'clock. We had to have time to get through check-in. We needed to be ready to board when our flight number was called.

We spent way over an hour trying to figure how in the hell we were going to get everything that we had picked up at the conference packed. We were only allowed two checked suitcases on the flight. We must have repacked those things more than 4 or 5 times before finally coming up with a solution.

It was too early in the morning for all of this activity and before breakfast too. I became extremely aggravated and frustrated as we kept working on it. We finally had no choice except to put our dirty laundry into one of the carry on bags, and then stack stuff and squeeze the rest of it into the two wheeled cases and the other carry on bag. All I could think as I tried to zip the suitcase, which wouldn't begin to close until I sat on it, was thank God it has wheels. I could almost feel the pain in my hips and lower back if I tried to pick that damn thing up and carry it for any length of time. It felt like it weighed a damn ton!

After getting dressed and having a cup of coffee in the room we went downstairs to join everyone else for the closing ceremonies of the conference. Nancy made a short speech before breakfast, outlining the preparation that had gone into planning the event. There had been the invitations sent out to the guest speakers, confirmation of their participation, organizing the menu and working with the staff of the hotel to provide not only the food, but the shuttle service to the participants, providing all of the snacks and refreshments during the breaks, and of course making sure that the sound system and program ran smoothly and stayed on schedule. She concluded by saying everyone should relax and enjoy a hearty breakfast before the ceremonies started.

The room was beautifully decorated with red and white balloons in the ceiling, and each table was set with crisp white linen table cloths and napkins, and had a bouquet of balloons in the center, tied with colorful ribbons with a weight attached, to hold them in place.

On each table was an assortment of Danishes, Muffins, Breakfast Breads, Croissants and Bagels with Cream Cheeses, Butter, Margarine, Preserves and Honey, Freshly Brewed Gourmet 100% Arabica Blend Coffee, Brewed Decaffeinated Coffee and International Assorted Teas. In the serving lines were freshly Squeezed Orange Juice, Tomato Juice, Cranberry Juice, Grapefruit Juice and Bottled Water. There was sliced fresh seasonal fruit and berries, assorted fruit yogurts, Individual Kellogg's cereals, skim and 2% milk, oatmeal,

Apple pancakes with Honey butter and warm maple syrup, house-made cheese blintzes with strawberry sauce and sour cream, Fluffy scrambled eggs, grilled half Roma tomatoes, spinach and mushrooms, hard boiled eggs, country sausage links, crispy bacon strips, and home fried breakfast potatoes.

As Barbara sat at the table we had chosen, I went up to get our breakfast because the lines were moving slowly, even though there were two. It was set up buffet-style so each person chose what they wanted and how much. I had to make a couple of trips back and forth to carry it all without having an accident. There was a family at our table who had traveled across the country to attend the event, and it was their daughter who was the survivor.

In the process of having the cancer in her mouth removed, she had also had to endure having her face reconstructed. Although she spoke softly when she had something to say, she had chosen not to eat breakfast. It turned out she was embarrassed because she drooled, due to the condition of her mouth when she ate. Barbara pointed that out no one in the room would pay attention to it, because we'd all been affected one way or the other, and besides, with all of the free food available, everyone was going to be too busy stuffing their faces to pay any attention. She ate breakfast, and thanked us several times for joining their table.

Some of us who were dealing with mouth issues ranging from sores to new dental work, or like myself who had to be careful what we ate, and had to chew slowly, were still enjoying the last remnants of the delicious food as the program got under way.

There was a survivor panel set up in the front that was made up of several of the SPOHNC chapter facilitators, survivors and a moderator.

They each gave an outline of their cancer battle, and then they took questions from members of the audience.

It was a very informative part of the program and I could tell that Barbara, although not physically taking notes with paper and pen (they had been packed), was making mental notes of the things that she would add to the ones she'd already taken, before typing a copy for the support group back home.

Dr. James J. Sciubba, DMD, PhD, past Director of Dental and Oral Medicine at Johns Hopkins Medicine and Vice President of SPOHNC gave a presentation on how far the organization had come in the 15 years that it had been in business, when Nancy started it at her house after she was diagnosed with mouth cancer, and wanting to talk with people who had dealt with it, could find no support groups in her area.

Everyone enjoyed the next part of the program tremendously. Norm Crosby, survivor (of throat cancer) and a comedian, who traveled across the country and performed in big nightclubs or casino's in places such as Las Vegas, put on a show.

It was stand-up comedy at it's best, and he incorporated some of his experiences with the disease into it, having those of us in the audience literally falling out of our chairs laughing, some with tears actually running down their cheeks.

The most touching and poignant part of the entire conference and celebration in my opinion, was near the end, before Nancy made the closing remarks.

It was a salute to all of the survivors in attendance who had dealt with, and come through treatment for oral head and neck cancer. Members of the SPOHNC staff and volunteers, had baskets of white and red carnations, and Nancy asked survivors to stand, according to the number of years they'd been survivors, and each was presented with one red and one white carnation.

Barbara had tears streaming down her cheeks as I stood up and was presented with my carnations and we took pictures of me holding them up. It might sound stupid to some people, but I was proud to be given those little flowers.

It meant I had faced the dragon, and through excellent medical care, a lot of heartache and pain, hard work and true grit and determination, had defeated it, and had refused to let it control me.

Nancy closed the conference with a short heart-felt speech about the success of the event, and thanking everyone who attended, wishing them the best in the endeavor to keep successfully moving forward. Barbara and I had the opportunity to wait up front to speak with Norm Crosby. He was just an ordinary guy who loved talking to people, and we had our picture taken with him to add to our collection of things from the trip.

We left the ballroom and gathering all of our stuff from the room went outside to wait for the shuttle bus to come back and take us to LaGuardia for our flight home. We got to say goodbye to several of the people we had spent time talking with and collected several addresses so we could write to each other.

It had been a very successful trip, but we were glad to be going home. I was just hoping that the flight back would be a safe and uneventful one, and I was looking forward to getting home. I had enjoyed the trip and learned so much I didn't know. It was a new experience for me. But now, as we were preparing to leave, I realized how much I had missed being at home.

From Flight to Fight

We went back to the room for our luggage and made sure we hadn't forgotten anything. There were a lot of bottled drinks that we had left on the Armoire that would be thrown away. We hated leaving them behind, but with such strict regulations at the airport, we didn't dare try taking them with us. We did grab one each to drink before we boarded the plane. We made our way downstairs and outside to the entrance to wait for the shuttle bus, after saying goodbye to the Assistant Manager behind the registration desk. We had the chance to say goodbye to several of the people we had talked to, including Dr. Rosenthal as he was leaving.

After waiting about forty-five minutes, we were finally able to board the shuttle for the airport. You could actually see the airport from the front entrance of the hotel, across in the distance. The driver who was operating the shuttle today wasn't the same one we had on Friday evening, and he wasn't as friendly or outgoing as his co-worker. He didn't have much to say at all as people boarded and found seats.

The streets of New York, at least the ones that we traveled on during the short time that we were there, definitely needed some major improvements done to them. They were more like washboards, with ruts so deep that it caused the bus to bounce up and down, tossing us from one side to the other, and several of the passengers grunted in frustration when their heads collided with the side of the bus. It didn't help much that the driver was speeding along like he was going to a fire, or that he seemed impatient to get rid of all of us. Barbara would swear when we got to the airport that her teeth rattled so much it was a wonder she hadn't heard them break.

La Guardia was so big and covered so much space, the shuttle made several stops for some of the other passengers to disembark at the location where they would check in for their flights. We were about the fourth or fifth stop, and as we left the shuttle, there was a mix-up about which luggage belonged to us. Thankfully, we were able to stop the driver and settle it before he darted off with the other passengers.

There were uniformed porters outside of the airport to help passengers find the location they needed, and once again the language barrier was very frustrating for us. We asked several of them for information as we tried to find out where we were supposed to go once we were inside the airport. They were either too busy to answer us or turned away, ignoring us altogether. I finally managed to get across the fact that I needed to find a wheelchair for Barbara so we could go inside for our flight.

A uniformed worker, a heavy-set young woman who looked very breathless finally arrived pushing one of the smallest chairs they had at the airport, and didn't give Barbara time to hardly sit down and get her feet up on the foot rests, before she took off pushing the chair through the wide automatic double doors.

We knew we had more than an hour before our flight was called, and were planning to get something cold to drink and use the restroom there at the airport before boarding the plane. The woman seemed to have an agenda all her own, and was determined to take us where she wanted us to go. Barbara finally got so disgusted and aggravated that she put her foot down and made her stop. The woman got real mad and turned around marching off in the same direction we had just come, mumbling under her breath.

After finding and using the bathroom, and buying a drink to share since they were so expensive, we made our way down a long steep ramp to the ground level where we had to sign in, get our boarding passes and wait for our flight number to be called over the intercom. I explained to them at the ticket counter that we needed someone to take Barbara to the plane because she was in the wheelchair.

Within several minutes after our flight had been called, two young girls in uniform, who looked no older than high school students, came down to take Barbara out to the plane. Instead of taking her out of one of the side doors on the side where we could see planes on the tarmac, they began pushing her back up the steep ramp. They were taking her out of one of the side doors farther up.

Evidently, neither of the girls were used to handling someone who was in a wheelchair, because even working together they couldn't seem to guide it in a straight line. They were weaving back and forth, almost hitting the wall and railing on one side.

There were two airline pilots walking down the ramp deep in conversation. To spare them from being run over with the chair, Barbara yelled out: Gang Way!! Looking up at the commotion, they immediately darted out of the way—and a good thing too, or they'd have been hit. It turned out one of them was the pilot for our plane, and he gave us thumbs up when we boarded.

The flight back was pretty uneventful, and both of us snoozed a little during the flight. I managed to stay awake longer than Barbara, who once we were in the air, settled back into a comfortable position and promptly dozed off. She didn't sleep long, and the flight went a little faster than scheduled because we had a good tailwind pushing us along.

When we arrived back in Charlottesville, there was a wheelchair waiting for us and we went almost immediately to the baggage claim area. We had two carry on bags each, and the two wheeled pieces that had been checked. When we got to the carousel, we only had one of the duffel bags and the smallest wheeled case.

The large one was missing, evidently not making it onto the plane at LaGuardia. Damn! Of all the incompetent—it was the main one we wanted, because in addition to our expensive dress clothing, it was where we'd packed all of the items and information we worked so hard to collect.

The porter was very apologetic and gave us the toll-free number to call. He said our luggage would be on the next flight coming in from New York later in the evening and we should call and make sure before driving back to the airport.

Barbara waited outside of the main entrance and watched our luggage while I walked to the parking lot and picked up the car, paying the attendant the parking fee.

The traffic was light and we made good time in driving from the airport home. We stopped for gas, cigarettes and something cold to drink before leaving town. When we got home we checked our mail, and had a box full in the three days since it had last been checked. Our answering machine had a lot of calls on it too.

After unloading the luggage and bringing it in, we changed into old comfortable clothes and I lay down to relaxed. Barbara headed to her computer to check all of the email she knew would be waiting.

Barbara called everyone to let them know we had gotten home safely, including Vikki. She called the toll-free number frequently, until finally exasperated by a recording; she finally gave up and called the airport.

She learned our luggage had arrived and it was behind the counter where it had been sitting since around eight that evening. I had already undressed and gone to bed for the night, so I had to get up, get dressed and drive back to the airport. I wasn't about to let it stay there overnight, afraid that it might disappear or be sent off on another trip to only God knew where.

It was such an honor for me that Vikki and the cancer center worked so hard for me and Barbara to go to New York for the conference and celebration, and to represent our small group of survivors and care givers at such a prestigious event.

We gained a lot of useful information from the key-note speakers, as well as talking with other survivors who had been where I was, and I heard about things that had helped them regain control over different areas of their lives affected by cancer. Since then, I have been able to overcome many obstacles of my own, although I still deal with some of them daily.

Novocaine Eases Pain

After we returned from our trip to New York we were still struggling financially, but we were both stubborn and determined that we weren't going to let it get the best of us. The benefits we were receiving from the Department of Social Services and from Social Security helped, but it certainly wasn't enough to cover all of our expenses.

Barbara and I had cut corners and expenses every way that we could think of and we still couldn't make the money stretch from one month until the next. We had run the entire spectrum of ideas to make extra money almost from the very first day I had been diagnosed.

We were busy cleaning and holding the yard sales every weekend which took a lot of time and hard work. Sometimes, when money was really tight or we had a bill that was definitely due, we would set one up during a week day down in Gordonsville. We were surprised that sometimes we did as good as or even better than when we had them on Saturday or Sunday.

I finally finished all of the chemotherapy and radiation treatments and the surgery, thank God, had been a success. I would still be kept on a five year watch list. According to my doctors, that was when a patient could and sometimes did, have a recurrence of the same cancer, or finds it has spread to another part of the body. Their word for that is metastasized. Too complicated for me; I'm a country boy who speaks plain English! For the moment, Dr. Reibel had assured me that I was cancer free; either way, I was a survivor.

Unfortunately, society doesn't see things quite the way we do. Whether it was because they were ignorant and uneducated or just didn't care is hard to say. I heard so many times while I was going through my treatments and even as I was regaining my strength: we wish you or we wish your husband a speedy recovery. A speedy recovery, what was that? There is nothing, not one thing speedy about recovering from cancer.

You never fully recover from it; you are a survivor with survivorship issues; issues that you have to deal with on a day to day basis for weeks, months, years and often times for the rest of your life. So what did they know? Speedy recovery, indeed!

Depending on the type of cancer a person was dealing with, the residual side affects could be mild, moderate and sometimes, severe. Life is never the same for us after the diagnosis. We always are searching for a "new normal", whatever that might be. We have to compensate for things we had that most people take for granted. It just aggravated the hell out of me when people would tell me that they wished me a speedy recovery. I'd bite my lip and tongue to keep from saying what I was thinking.

I had been very fortunate that I had overcome so many eating challenges that I had faced when I was going through my treatments. I had swallowing and chewing issues to deal with, and often compensated my shortcomings by using the chopper or the blender, and drinking a lot of the Ensure and Carnation Instant Breakfast products. Now, with all of that behind me, I would once again be confronted with dealing with nutritional problems.

Instead of complications of treatments, this time the culprit was changes that were going on inside my mouth. While the chemotherapy and radiation had been instrumental in helping successfully overcoming the cancer, it had literally destroyed a lot of my gum line and the bone structure inside of my mouth. Added with the fact that I also suffered with periodontal disease that is hereditary in my family, it was a major contributor to my having to have all of my permanent teeth removed. I was very upset and depressed when my dentist gave me this news.

I had been certain that with all of the fluoride trays and treatments I had used, the cavities that had been filled and the maintenance program that I was using every day would be enough to protect my teeth and save them. I thought everything was going smoothly, because I had always received good reports when I visited my dentist.

The first thing that popped into my head was what would I look like without my teeth and just how the hell was I supposed to be able to eat. I certainly couldn't imagine going about my daily routine without my teeth. NO! Hadn't I already been through enough? Suffered enough embarrassment? I'd felt useless as I recovered—like the world was out to get me at times. Like things seemed to move along without me, and now I had to go through this too? When would it ever end?

Another major problem was since we were literally at the bottom of the barrel financially, how in the world we were going to be able to come up with hundreds, if not a thousand dollars, to pay for dentures for me? I had so many questions and it looked as if there weren't going to be any easy answers to any of them. But I had one major hurdle to get through before the teeth would become an issue.

My dentist, Dr. Grimm, scheduled an appointment for me in the Hyperbaric Clinic located in the main hospital. Hyperbaric is pressurized oxygen delivered as you are lying in a sealed chamber, and is very similar to that of an MRI Machine. Well! I didn't particularly enjoy being in an elevator, so I wondered how I would deal with being inside of that machine. It was going to be tough, especially knowing that I couldn't get out until the person in charge depressurized and unlocked it.

The chamber itself is round—like a large cylinder, see-through so that the staff of the clinic can monitor you while you are inside, and also keep a check on your vital signs throughout the treatment. There is a small bed (smaller than the ones used in exam rooms or clinics that slides up inside of the chamber on rollers.

The patient is asked to undress and put on booties and a standard hospital gown for comfort. The pressurized oxygen is cold after you are exposed to it for several minutes so they also provide you with a heavy sheet to cover up.

I wasn't exactly thrilled about being placed inside of that sealed compartment and to help me relax, Dr. Reibel prescribed Adavan that I was to take approximately thirty minutes before my scheduled appointment. Sometimes the medication worked pretty well, and there were days that it didn't.

I would either close my eyes and try to "nap" just to shut out the fact I was sealed inside; trying to put it out of my mind. One of the staff usually sat in a chair beside the tank, reading or doing paperwork, checking on me every few minutes, asking a question or two, or reminding me when it was time to breathe into the oxygen mask beside me on the bed.

I would also watch television sometimes since there was one mounted on the wall right outside the chamber, and they would pipe the sound inside to me. I watched a lot of Matlock with Andy Griffith and Judging Amy episodes. Every now and then for variety I would get to see little House on the Prairie.

Altogether I would have to take twenty treatments during the first round of the Hyperbaric and each one of the treatments lasted about two hours. Barbara went with me to one of them and I will never forget the reaction she had to seeing me lying inside of that chamber.

When we left the house, she had put a packet of blank Christmas cards and envelopes along with addresses for some of the soldiers stationed in Iraq that she had become pen pals with, into her purse. She said that they would keep her busy while I was getting my treatment and she would wait for me in the waiting room.

I didn't need to register downstairs for the treatments and went on to the clinic. We stopped by the waiting room where she would stay. There was a table in the middle of the room and Barbara sat down at it as the nurse came through the door to take me back to the treatment area. About 45 minutes later, once I had changed into the hospital gown and the treatment started, I asked the nurse if she would ask Barbara if she would like to come in and sit with me. I had the use of a microphone and we could at least talk to each other.

When she came into the room and got her first look at me inside the machine her face turned chalk white and she collapsed into the chair that was beside it, not saying a word for several seconds.

She is extremely claustrophobic and can't deal with tightly closed or dark places. One time she had to be taken out of a scheduled MRI for her back because she had been unable to breathe. Now I could see her body shaking, like she was shivering because she was very cold. She sat there for about five minutes, and then she told me she couldn't stay in there with me, and made a beeline for the door. She went back to the waiting room and actually burst into tears as she walked in, prompting the lady working at the information desk to ask if she was alright. She asked if Barbara wanted her to call someone for her

A few minutes later, she managed to pull herself together by going to the bathroom and washing her face with cold water. From that day on I went to the treatments but she stayed at home and we never talked about them. Once I finished the twentieth treatment, I had to wait for ten days to get an appointment with the dental clinic.

I had been faithful about keeping all of my appointments and I didn't like some of them but I managed without too much problem, to get through them. This is one that I dreaded going to and as each day went by and the appointment got closer and closer, I became more agitated and moody. Finally, it was time to face the music.

I got to the clinic a few minutes early and registered at the desk before having a seat in the waiting room that was quite busy today. When they called me back to the office, my feet felt like I had lead in my shoes as I slowly put one foot in front of the other to follow the nurse. As I settled down into the chair, I was still having a hard time dealing with the fact I was going to lose my teeth. It just seemed so unfair to me that a treatment to cure one illness would cause so much devastation with another part of your body.

I had no idea what my initial reaction would be once Dr. Grimm finished taking my teeth, and I worried about what people would think when they saw me without them. I know it sounds vain, but I had never dealt with anything like this before. I wear a full beard, which thankfully since my treatments had ended had started filling out again, but I knew that it made my face look skinnier and longer than normal and I supposed it would be even worse without teeth and that bothered me too.

A few minutes after I'd been put into the chair with the blue paper bib clipped securely in place around my neck, Dr. Grimm and his assistant came into the room. I was nervous and fidgety and he tried to reassure me that he would be giving me enough Nova Cain to keep me from feeling anything except pressure. "Now, where have I heard that before," I wondered.

He put on the latex plastic gloves and had me open my mouth as wide as I could get it (which wasn't very much since the radiation had affected the range of motion in my jaw), and ran his index finger along my gum line as his assistant handed him the first needle.

I closed my eyes, jumping and flinching as the sharp end penetrated tender gums. "Oh, oh, oh', I grunted as the needle went deeper and deeper until he finally dislodged it. He gave my jaw a couple of tugs as he laid the used needle and pump to the side on the little metal tray. Assuring me that he would give the medicine time to start working, he began gathering the rest of his instruments, and was reading my chart and x-rays.

Even though the Nova cane began to work and my gums were indeed numb, I felt every one of the following needles that were inserted. If not physically, then emotionally as it brought me closer and closer to the reality that when it was over, and I got up out of the chair I was leaving behind my teeth.

I had no idea what difficulties I would face, other than I was losing another part of myself because of a disease that had literally turned my life and world inside out and upside down. The problems seemed to be insurmountable to me at times. All during the remainder of that visit, with each tug Dr. Grimm made, I felt the pressure physically and emotionally and I tried to keep my eyes closed as a feeling of despair and depression threatened to overwhelm me.

I left the clinic over an hour later, with my mouth bleeding profusely and my mouth packed with gauze. I had to make several stops along the road on the way home to change it and to spit, to keep the blood from sliding into my throat. My face remained numb for about 3 hours and it was hard opening my mouth to change the gauze because it was so swollen.

Dr. Grimm had written me a prescription for pain medication which I had filled at the pharmacy before leaving, and I was truly grateful for it when the nova cane began to wear off. After removing my teeth there were several places in my gums where he had to put in stitches because some of the teeth had such deep long roots that it left gaping holes where the teeth had been.

For the next four days I could only manage to eat things that were room temperature and nothing that was hot. It caused too much pain to my tender gums. He had given me a syringe with a crooked tip so that I could apply warm salt water to the back areas, and use the oral antiseptic rinse he had prescribed before bed.

It took about two weeks for my gums to heal enough that he could remove the stitches. Once he was satisfied that I didn't contract any sort of infection, he set an appointment for me to come in to have the bottom teeth removed. The whole process was very challenging for me. It not only affected me in the physical sense, but emotionally. I mean, hey,

I'm only human. It is a major adjustment for someone to go through when they lose their teeth.

I had to wait for a couple of weeks to let my bottom gums heal a little before Dr. Grimm sent me to the Hyperbaric Clinic to finish the last ten treatments of the pressurized oxygen. It would actually help prevent any further complications and speed up the healing process. It would still be a long wait before Dr. Grimm would start to consider preparing me for dentures. He already warned me that it wouldn't happen overnight. But I wondered just how long I would really have to wait.

It was approximately ten months later, during one of my routine checkups that he explained the process. In order for a set of dentures to be made for me he would need to do a complete series of dental molds with wait periods in between each set. With the amount of bone loss and the deterioration of my gum line, it was the only way to insure a good fit. He estimated that the total time would be somewhere around three months.

When I went in to the clinic to have the second mold made, I was approached by the Manager of the clinic about how I was planning to pay for the dentures. The total cost for them was $450.00. I had known I would have to face this hurdle, and had no clue on where I would find the money to pay for them. With both Barbara and I on Social Security, and the income from the yard sales no longer coming in, the only choice I had was to sit down with Vikki Bravo and see if she could help me find a resource. I was surprised that there was something called the Hope Fund at the University. It had been established in honor of a breast cancer survivor, who had worked as a volunteer, and its purpose was to help cancer patients with expenses such as utility bills, dentures, etc. There was a $400 limit, and she said that she would talk to the manager of the Dental Clinic after she received confirmation from the Hope Fund After all of the arrangements, my final out-of-pocket cost was $50, that they allowed me to pay in two installments.

The next hurdle that I would have to deal with would prove to be the longest and most aggravating one of all. How was I going to be able to eat now that my teeth had been removed? My gums were soft and very tender, and just the thought of trying to chew with them made me shudder and shake my head. I thought that I had solved all of the problems with nutrition I would have to deal with after the radiation and chemotherapy. With my weight already being a problem, what would happen now that I would have a hard time eating just about anything?

Barbara and I soon discovered that the chopper and blender was a constant friend, but that it was also an enemy. Everything I put into my mouth had to be chopped like baby food or pureed until it was liquefied. The problem was having the money to buy the food to chop or puree.

Without the income from the yard sales coming in weekly, we were back to pinching pennies. I needed to eat fresh fruits and vegetables, pastas, a lot of dairy products and meats that would help to replenish my body with all of the nutrients that had been depleted as the result of the chemotherapy and radiation.

The real question was where was the money going to come from to pay for it? I had no answer to the question. It was a given fact that we couldn't rely on Social Services and the Food Stamp Program because they had already determined that according to their guidelines, we had too much income, and were eligible for only $10 a month in assistance. Can you believe that? It had certainly taken us by complete surprise. The problem with that program was that they don't count all of the bills the applicant has to pay out of whatever source of income that they have coming into the household. They count rent and utility bills, basic telephone service, and any out-of-pocket medical expenses. Ok. That is understandable. In my particular case, they also counted the lot rent since we live in a mobile home park. Cool. But wait a minute; what about the other bills? I mean, come on. People have car payments, car insurance, gas, car maintenance, house supplies, cable bills (if they want to keep up with the outside world), clothing, and food. Not counting these bills just didn't make any sense.

We quickly learned that in the Commonwealth of Virginia, there are no nutritional programs to help indigent or low income families with special nutritional needs other than the Food Stamp Program or area Food Banks. I think the Food Banks are a wonderful resource, and applaud them for all that they do to help families in need. However, with only canned and prepackaged foods available from them it would not meet the nutrient rich foods my body needed. Where would I be able to find help with those things?

Barbara was constantly on the telephone and the computer, sometimes for hours at a time trying to find a suitable solution for this problem, and never found any satisfactory results. Every time she turned around she had one door after another slammed in her face. Not just here locally in our community either. She called national and regional organizations—one who claimed to help cancer patients and you know what? The only thing all of them suggested to her was to call Social Services and the Food Banks.

Thankfully, through pure grit and determination, she managed to locate one or two of the churches within our community that offered assistance with food coupons to area stores such as Food Lion and

Kroger, and one who gave us five boxes of food—including meats, dairy and perishable products we were able to divide and freeze for future meals or casseroles to make it last.

One church in Albemarle County was a God send. The pastor Bill Love said that he would help us out with a few groceries to tide us over. He went to Sam's Club and bought meats, eggs, milk, cereals, fruits and vegetables in bulk—fresh and frozen that helped us out tremendously

An owner of a local newspaper in Charlottesville stepped in and we were blessed with more help when she went shopping for us at Food Lion after asking Barbara to make a list of needed items and sending it to her by email. I drove over to the Food Lion in the Forest Lakes Shopping Center on Route 29 and was amazed at the amount of food she had purchased. There was some that Barbara said wasn't on the list she had emailed.

When my dentures were finally ready, I went in to pick them up. Dr. Grimm told me because of the amount of bone that had been destroyed; my dentures would never have a tight, secure fit. The only way I would ever get a tight fit was to use a denture adhesive.

I wondered how many more products I was going to have to adjust to as I searched for a new "normal" every survivor I had met to date kept referring to. I was already trying every product on the market to deal with dry mouth. I was always looking in pharmacies and stores when we went shopping to see if there was anything I hadn't tried.

Here my dentist, after all of the mold fittings to ensure a "proper" fit was telling me that I'd never have it. And would have to use some nasty cream or power on the denture to hold it in? Damn! How many more things was I going to have to adjust to and work on to get right for myself? It kept getting harder and harder to keep a positive attitude.

I have found since then, that it is not only a nuisance to use these products; the ooze can be uncontrollable, often coming out into my mouth once the dentures are in place, but it is very time consuming as well. I have had the dentures for almost a year now, and I am still very self-conscious with them. I think that my speech is very different when I am wearing them, and often feel like people have a hard time understanding me when I talk to them.

I am not comfortable going out into public places such as events or restaurants to eat, because I am afraid that the denture adhesive will stop working and they will become loose while I am chewing or even talking.

Breaking News

Barbara had become very frustrated with all of the organizations that were designed to help cancer patients and didn't. At the top of the list was ACS—the American Cancer Society, who's Regional Director admitted during a telephone conversation that they didn't have a program to meet the nutritional needs patients found themselves facing. Well that made no sense. As much money as they had given to them every year, all of the Relays for Life, and fundraisers they had. Where was the money going? Printing all of the pamphlets that people needed a college degree or dictionary to understand? Or to pay for the multi-billion dollar research facility they had in Texas? It sure as hell wasn't helping those of us who needed it the most.

She wanted to do something to make the public aware of what cancer patients had to deal with from diagnosis and especially as they received the treatments and then moved forward into dealing with survivorship issues. She spent days on the telephone talking to the local television stations about doing a story, and for what?

You would think that they would be willing to help provide assistance by bringing it to their viewer's attention; to get it out there and help make a difference. They reported so much bad news each and every day. What about a human interest story that would have a positive impact? Surely they would jump at a chance to put that on their program. But NO! Each and every one of them flat refused to become involved. I found it so hard to believe. They will report rape, murder, gang related news, local, state and national political news, stories about how agencies help those in need, but they can't do a story on the problems of a cancer patient? Of course they can't. They all were too concerned about other organizations and people who might need their help too, and it would mean hard work or maybe overtime. But yet they were winning awards for excellence. Bah! The people who gave those awards needed their heads examined if you ask me.

Now they had done it! They had Barbara steaming mad with that attitude. And I wasn't far behind her! Come on people, can't somebody give me a break for once? Determined not to give up, Barbara called our local daily paper and spoke with one of the reporters there, Bryan McKenzie. Bryan had been writing a column for the paper for years, and his specialty was human interest and people stories, not gossipy ones like the tabloids.

The reason she wanted to do an interview and article was to bring to light that, while cancer patients may now be listed as "survivors", their battle had only just begun. The issues and all of the complications, the side effects and how the disease impacted and changed everything in their lives, was devastating and needed to be understood.

When she talked about her idea with Bryan, he agreed to come out and sit down with us and talk to figure out how he could help. He drove out for a visit, taking a lot of notes as we explained all of the problems I had been through, things I was still dealing with and some of the things we had done in order to be able to survive so far: the donation jars, yard sales, relying on churches and friends.

He wrote a very informative article which he titled "Surviving Wolves at the Door." We were quite frankly stunned by the reader's response to that article. It was nothing like we had anticipated.

We didn't do the article for financial gain. It never entered our thoughts. All we wanted was to make the public aware of cancer and its horrifying effect on a person's life. We never thought we would get anything out of it personally. However, we received food vouchers to Food Lion, gift cards from different organizations, checks from people in Albemarle, Charlottesville and Greene Counties, boxes of food from area churches, and one reader called Bryan and got the account number for our electric company, and paid our bill.

We were shocked and amazed at their generosity. Barbara, in an effort to take advantage of as much media exposure as was possible to bring awareness to cancer patients and survivors, called the weekly newspaper where we live, The Orange County Review.

She spoke with the editor, Jeffrey Poole. When she explained what she wanted to do, Mr. Poole suggested she write a letter to the editor, so he could read over it before deciding the best way route to take. Barbara emailed him over the internet and also sent him a copy in the mail. Two weeks later, she called him back to find out what, if anything, he had to suggest.

He said that he had hired a new reporter, but that it would be several weeks before he would be free to do a story. Barbara was hopeful that once the reporter got adjusted at the paper that he would call and be willing to come out and write another story. It would reach people that perhaps the article in the other paper had missed, and it just might make a difference.

The reporter, John Hooten, came out to the house and did an in-depth interview; asking about all of the treatments, what we did to survive paying bills and eventually also talked with Vikki Bravo before writing the story. Vikki was able to confirm everything we told him and that went a long way as far as credibility. He took a picture of me sitting in my kitchen to put with the story, and was gracious enough to send several copies to share with all of the organizations that we are involved in and to have a copy for our scrapbook and resources.

This doesn't really pertain to a NEWSPAPER article, but a support group newsletter, but it was still news right?

George Visich, a member of our support group who is a long time survivor of cancer and a laryngectomee, is very active in talking with area school children about the dangers of smoking and has been working with the American Cancer Society and their Relay for Life for years.

His daughter, Rosemarie Lanard is a Vice President for the investment firm of Standard and Poole in New York City. She lives in Connecticut with her family, and because her dad is a group member she subscribes to the monthly newsletter via email.

The writer of the news letter, also another survivor would include things about Barbara and me: we were looking for donations for our yard sales, etc. And he mentioned us quite often!

She mailed Vikki an envelope for us and Vikki called and wanted to know if I could pick it up that afternoon when I came in to go to work. Vikki had taken it home with her the night before, so we figured it must be important, so we told her that we would come over the next morning early and get it.

When we got over there as usual, it was a nightmare trying to find a parking space at Hospital West. I let Barbara out at the front door since we were bringing Vikki a bag of clothing we had for her, and she went in to page her while I kept driving around looking for a parking space.

By the time I finally managed to locate and make it to the front entrance, Barbara had talked to Vikki, and was sitting on one of the wooden benches outside. She had a business-size envelope clutched tightly in her hand, and I could tell something had upset her when I looked at her face.

There were tear tracks on her face and I asked her what was wrong. She said she would tell me when we got to the car, and stood up. I took the envelope, and glancing inside, my eyes widened in shock. There was a lot of money in it and I saw twenty dollar bills.

When we got in the car and Barbara counted it, we both cried. There was FIVE HUNDRED DOLLARS in it, all in twenties; along with a note that said she hoped this would help and that if we needed anything else to be sure to let her know. We couldn't believe it! Why would a stranger (even if her dad was in our support group) be so generous to us? It was mind-boggling.

What Did You Say?

One thing has constantly amazed and confused me at the same time. During the time I've spent in treatment and recovery, the negative responses we as survivors and patients receive are a travesty. It is especially hard to swallow when it comes from our elected officials and people who work for them. I mean, come on. These are the very folks we expect to be on our side—after all, it was our trust and votes which put them into their positions and gave them the authority they have.

There was one particular incident that sticks out in my mind like a sore thumb, because it came from the one place where we had least expected it. Of course, now looking back I suppose we should have known better than to contact them anyway. But then again, desperate situations call for desperate measures, or so I've heard.

Barbara tried so hard to find help for our food crisis, and was really worried about me more than she was for herself. She spent days making calls and getting absolutely nowhere with the system. Having run out of places to call she decided to place a call to one of the legislative assistants in the Governor's office. She wanted to find out if perhaps he or she would know of some program that could help, that she had somehow overlooked. She never had the opportunity to speak with the Assistant.

When the switchboard operator for the Governor's office answered the phone, Barbara explained that I was a cancer survivor who, because of radiation had to have all of my teeth removed, and had lost 45 pounds during treatment and that I needed fresh fruits, vegetables and meats, and that on our limited income of Social Security disability we had no money left to purchase the food, and didn't qualify for help from the Department of Social Services. She told the operator that she wished to speak to one of the Governor's legislative assistants about the problem.

The operator never switched her call to the legislative assistant. She became very obnoxious, even arrogant in her attitude toward Barbara. She told her that she had no suggestions to make other than my wife should use the internet and the Google Search Engine to start up a non-profit organization to meet our needs. I was sitting in the chair in the living room getting ready to do my exercise program, and I will never forget the expression on Barbara's face. It went from shock to anger in the space of a split second, and her face was so red I thought it would burst into flames any second. And then she told me what the woman had said to her.

Excuse me? What did she say? Why, of all the stupid, hair brained things—who in the hell—start a non profit organization, when we barely had two nickels to rub together. Who was she kidding? Before I could say one word, Barbara went off.

I mean she completely lost all grip on her temper, which was already strained, and very quickly informed her "I don't know what planet you dropped to earth from, but they need to beam your ass back there quick, because if I had the money to start a non-profit organization, why in the hell would I be calling you in the first place? Then she very promptly slammed the phone down in her ear. She was so mad she was literally shaking and I couldn't blame her. I had never heard such a stupid thing in all my life.

I know you're probably thinking my wife should have kept her cool and not made that comment to the woman. Under normal circumstances, Barbara would have ignored it and hung up without ever saying a word. It's not always that easy.

When you are fighting for everything you need, it is very frustrating. But when, every time you turn around, you get one negative, and yes, even stupid comments made, it can be too much. They brush you off like you're not important. After a while it begins to get to you deep down inside, like you don't feel bad enough to have to ask for help. You get the courage up to ask and then get shot down with idiotic responses

Barbara had been the one who had to take care of all of the business affairs, dealing with everything from paying the bills, talking with creditors, handling all of my appointments, treatments, medication changes, refills and the constant barrage of telephone calls, on top of taking care of my physical, nutritional and emotional needs since I'd been diagnosed.

A person can only handle so much stress before something has to give. Under the circumstances, I applaud her for standing up and speaking her mind. The woman, a representative of the Governor, had no right to take such a rude and obnoxious attitude with someone who called looking for help.

One evening several weeks later, after all of the work for the day had been done, I was relaxing in my recliner in the living room watching television. Barbara was sitting at the kitchen table enjoying a cup of coffee and glancing through some of the materials we had picked up on the trip to New York.

She found the address for the Lance Armstrong Foundation, and had a thought. Since he was working to improve quality care for cancer patients, why not write him a letter. She quickly grabbed some paper and pen and started one. She told him my story without going into a lot of detail: about the struggles and problems we had been encountering, the attitudes of the people and the things we needed and couldn't afford. She never really expected to get any type of response from him. I think that at this point she did it just to get all of the anger and frustration out of her system.

Late one afternoon, about five days later, the telephone rang, and when Barbara answered, the Special Projects Manager from the Lance Armstrong Foundation was calling in reference to her letter. We sat there in stunned silence, our mouths hanging open as we listened to her talk. We automatically responded to the questions about treatment, and the options we had tried.

After gathering all of the information she needed, she told Barbara she was going to refer our file to a case manager who would be calling to follow up with us on the issues we'd discussed. Several days later, we received a call from the case manager.

We worked with her on a couple of different occasions, and were able to apply for, and receive a small stipend check issued from the Patient Advocate Foundation located in Newport News, Virginia. The stipend was actually provided through a grant funded by the Lance Armstrong Foundation. It was designated to help patients like me, who had received and completed all of their treatments. However, even with the treatments behind them, they had financial needs they weren't able to meet without some type of assistance. We finally received the check from them about three weeks later for one hundred and twenty-five dollars. It may sound like a small amount to you, but it meant the world to us.

The lady was also kind enough to refer us to another case manager at the Patient Advocate Foundation, Tammy Niece who was the program coordinator. She was able to help me obtain a rehabilitative device I needed for range of motion exercises for my jaw. Due to radiation, it had become stiff and I was unable to open it normally, without pain shooting throughout my entire face

The device, called a Therabyte, had been suggested by Dr. Grimm in the Dental Clinic and Dr. Read, in Radiology/Oncology. Unfortunately, Medicare didn't cover all of the expense, and I had not yet met my yearly deductible. I also did not have the money to pay my percentage of the cost.

Tammy Niece wrote a letter to the Ruritan Club in Barboursville Virginia asking if they would be willing to help us purchase the device.

After their monthly meeting, they sent us a letter to say that they were paying for it and that a check had been sent directly to the company. I received the device by UPS about three weeks later.

A Call to Action

Through persistence and overcoming a lot of negativity, we managed to get a lot of different things accomplished, and yet there had to be a way to tap into better quality care, better resources for patients and a way to deal with people, especially elected officials, in a more positive and structured way.

But where did you start? Was there actually a place out there that combined all of these qualities, and who worked toward making a difference, especially for people struck with such a debilitating and chronic disease such as cancer?

By this time Barbara was totally frustrated and disillusioned with the healthcare and private sector organizations. They didn't offer very much of the help needed by cancer patients. She began searching for other ways to make a difference.

Whenever she went with me to appointments at the Cancer Center, she would spend the time looking at different materials available and would gather the ones that her attention and bring them home. One morning as I was doing my exercises, she was sitting at the computer looking at some of the most recent pamphlets and brochures she had picked up.

She noticed a website (www.canceradvocacynow.org) and telephone number (1-888-650-9127) for the National Coalition for

Cancer Survivorship. Firing up her computer, she went online to the website to check it out.

One of the words that jumped off of the page at her was ADVOCACY. Impressed with the information on the website, she decided to call to find out more about how she could get involved with the work they were doing.

The organization, located in Silver Spring, Maryland is the oldest survivor-led organization in the United States and has been in operation since 1986 when it was founded in Albuquerque, New Mexico.

By putting the cancer patient first, the organization quickly earned the reputation of the "go to source" for information ranging from physical to psychological and spiritual needs.

In 1992 it relocated to its current location to be closer to the organizations and government agencies it worked with. Most of the staff of the diverse group are cancer survivors or have had a personal experience with the disease.

After reading all of the information on the website, she called the toll-free number to speak with someone about getting involved. She had a difficult time at first reaching the grassroots legislative part of the organization. She was eventually able to speak with Mark Gorman.

She gave her name and where she was calling from, and a brief outline of my cancer diagnosis, treatments and the side effects I was still dealing with. Then they talked about the problems we had to deal with on a daily basis, and some of the reactions of the people she had turned to for help.

She told him she was looking for a way to use our experiences in a positive way to help other cancer patients and survivors.

First, Mark suggested she go to their website and click on the action tab to register with their website. It would send alerts when there were important legislative issues that needed her Representatives attention, and their group would send a letter she could sign and send to Washington asking for her Representative's support.

Next, he suggested that she view the training module on the website about how to become an effective advocate.

When Barbara hung up after talking to Mark, she listened to the training module, and impressed, decided she definitely wanted to get involved.

She called Vikki at the cancer center and told her about what she had learned, and asked if she thought that some of the other patients and their families would be interested in learning about advocacy. Vikki was enthusiastic and said it sounded good, but since the group was involved in politics, she would need to find out if it was something that would be allowed at the cancer center.

She asked Barbara if the group did live trainings, and Barbara didn't know. She volunteered to call Mark Gorman back and to ask.

When she did, Mark said that he would be glad to come to Charlottesville to do a training session if she and Vikki thought that there would be enough interest to hold one. He said to talk it over together, and when she had more information let him know, and they could work on scheduling one

A Sensational Woman

In late February 2007, Barbara sat down at her computer, and using the Microsoft Word Program, began writing about some of the things we found through personal trial and error to have worked for us when figuring different issues of cancer: the diagnosis, dealing with finances, problems with food, money saving ideas, how to deal with Social Services the applications a person with cancer can fill out for assistance, how to deal with Social Security, and many other tidbits of information people might find valuable. When she finished the document, she emailed a copy of it to both Vikki Bravo and Diane Cole at the Cancer Center to see what their opinion of it was.

Diane was impressed with it and thought that it was a great resource that should be shared with the patients and their families, and asked Barbara if she could do a little editing on it to make it more reader friendly. Barbara, glad the document might be helpful, told her to do whatever she needed to improve it for them.

Barbara had also sent a copy of it to Ellen Desper, R.N. at the ENT Clinic who was very enthusiastic and told her that she would definitely put copies of it out for the patients that came into the clinic.

In March of 2007, Second Wind celebrated its 11th Anniversary and we were privileged to have Nancy Leupold, Founder and President of SPOHNC, who joined us for the celebration. Second Wind is a charter member of the national organization.

When we applied for membership, all of the work had been done via email, fax or over the telephone, so none of our members had ever had the privilege of meeting Nancy in person. Nancy also had never had the opportunity to visit the Charlottesville Virginia area.

She has a plate full: often working long, hard demanding, and often stressful hours Nancy is definitely a hands-on person and makes most of the day to day decisions on how things are done in the organization.

She travels extensively, going to seminars and conferences in addition working on the newsletter that is published nine times per year.

She is also a member of the board of many cancer related organizations. She applies for grants and spear-heads projects such as the cookbooks and the other publications that are offered by the organization, and along with the Webmaster, chooses the information included on their website at www.spohnc.org.

Vikki and Barbara discussed the idea of how wonderful it would be if they could have Nancy come to one of the groups celebrations and Barbara, wanting to help because she understood how demanding and time consuming Vikki's job was, offered to telephone SPOHNC and find out if it would be possible.

Nancy lives in Long Island, New York but spends her winter vacation in Florida. As luck would have it, in March, during our celebration, she would be leaving Florida to return home.

Nancy told Barbara that she would be delighted to come via Charlottesville, to pay a visit to one of her chapters. To accommodate Nancy's travel schedule, Vikki moved the meeting up one week so it would be held on the day of her arrival.

Our meetings are usually held at the Fontaine Research Park, in the Forestry Building. We were unsure of how many people would welcome the opportunity to attend the meeting with Nancy. Vikki moved the meeting to Hospital West on the 6th floor of the cancer center. We used the large board room and that gave us a place in the hallway to set up the buffet lunch.

Vikki suggested Barbara ask Nancy if the Cancer Center would receive a discount if they ordered multiple copies of the cookbook— Eat Well, Stay Nourished that SPOHNC had available at the Conference in New York.

Barbara had brought a copy back to share and several people in the group were interested in it. Nancy said that they would receive the discount and said she would be glad to bring the books with her when she came.

Barbara was in Vikki's office down from the boardroom making copies of the resource guide and other information to include in a notebook that she was planning on giving Nancy, when she and her husband arrived. She spoke to me and Barbara like we were old friends when we eventually joined her. It was good to see her again.

After a great lunch provided by the Biltmore Grille, Nancy gave an overview of SPOHNC and it had come into existence so many years before.

She had been diagnosed with cancer of the mouth and was searching for someone who had gone through the same diagnosis and treatment that she was now facing. She was shocked that there were no support groups available in her area. She eventually established the group, with help from experienced medical professionals some who would eventually become board members, out of a spare bedroom in her house.

Today, the organization has 55 chapters spread throughout the United States, and its website also includes a Volunteer Network. Barbara and I are registered with the Network as Survivor and Caregiver volunteers. The website is a great source of information, and it is constantly updated to meet the changing needs of patients, survivors and their families.

Vikki had a Certificate of Appreciation made and framed for Nancy, and had asked Larry Haywood, as the oldest member of the group (from the first meeting that was held) to present it to her.

We were able to take pictures of the moment to include in the groups photo album. (We are planning on getting a copy made and to buy a special frame for it before sending it on to Nancy).

When Nancy was ready to leave Barbara presented her with a copy of the Resource Guide she had put together back in February and some other information on products and services she thought that SPOHNC could use when people called in looking for assistance for different problems they were dealing with.

Since then, Nancy has asked her permission to include a lot of the information in a book that SPOHNC is putting together, written by other patients and caregivers, and which hopefully will be ready for distribution sometime in the spring of 2008. Shocked that Nancy wanted to use what she had written, Barbara gave her permission.

FULL STEAM AHEAD

In April 2007, Barbara and Vikki again talked about the idea of the advocacy training program, and Barbara was able to share how using the training manual in her letter writing campaign had made a difference in the responses she received back. She told Vikki that she really believed that it would be a worth while venture to have the program at the University.

Before any of that happened, the entire Second Wind group and a lot of staff with the cancer center had something planned for Vikki that she didn't have any idea was coming.

For a couple of months prior to the April meeting,, Gordon Putnam who is the Chaplain, and Barbara worked to send out notices in the newsletter, talked with staff at the cancer center and the different clinics, for donations towards getting a gift certificate to Vikki's favorite French Restaurant. We were also going to present her with a certificate of appreciation for everything she did in her job. Some of the things went well above and beyond what her job description called for.

We just thought that it would be nice to let her know how much she meant to us as a group and also as individuals, because she at times was our lifeline and helped us to stay grounded. The initial idea had been mine and Barbara's but everyone else was very enthusiastic about it. We came up with the idea when we got to see how she interacted with so many of the patients and survivors on our trips to the cancer center.

Gordon was on a business trip to San Francisco for a convention when the April meeting was held, and Barbara was the one who presented Vikki with the Certificate to her favorite restaurant that both she and her husband, Jerry could share. Barbara asked Larry Haywood to present the certificate of appreciation to her. Diane Cole, who had come to the meeting and had brought the certificates with her played photographer, using Barbara's digital camera to record the moment.

Vikki was absolutely shocked when they were presented to her. She had misty eyes as she accepted them, and became a little choked up as she thanked everyone for giving them to her. It was a very touching moment for those of us who love and depend on her for our source of inspiration and wisdom.

After that meeting, things would become very busy and hectic over the next several months. There were many projects and events that would be taking place, and once again, the project to bring advocacy to UVA was in the forefront.

Vikki took the issue of the advocacy program to Diane Cole the Manager of the cancer center for her opinion on the program. Diane was very enthusiastic about it and said it was definitely a program that they should look into providing for patients and their families. It would give them a way they would feel useful as well as having a way and to contribute and make a difference. Before we could receive the final go ahead, however, she would need to get final approval from sources higher up the chain of command with the University.

NCCS was affiliated with government and politics and the University was a state funded facility. It would be several months, and a lot of planning and hard work before the training could take place. In the meantime, Mark sent Barbara a copy of the training manual that

NCCS had put together. She began using it right away in the letter campaign which she had been working on for months prior to getting in touch with Mark the first time.

She had already written letters to most of the Virginia Delegation in Washington, including Senator John Warner, Senator James Webb and Congressman Eric Cantor. She had also gone so far as to write one to President George W. Bush! On the state level she had written to Senator Creigh Deeds, Senator Edd Houck and Delegate Robert Bell. She had received responses from Senator Deeds, and Edd Houck (written and email), and two responses from Delegate Robert Bell.

Her letters sometimes were long, running into two pages with all of the information she included. Using the training manual, she was able to write shorter, more effective letters and learned how to telephone the officials as well.

The idea of the cancer advocacy training program was still on, but put on hold while Vikki and her husband went on vacation in May, traveling to Israel for three weeks. Once Vikki returned, she was ready to begin the planning, and since Barbara was already working with Mark, she asked her to be the liaison and coordinate the program.

The telephone lines between Barboursville VA and Silver Spring Maryland buzzed and rang for days on end with calls traveling both ways, emails zipped back and forth between Mark and Barbara, and a lot of strategy planning, opinions and attention to small details were happening in order to put the program together.

Mark, at Barbara's request, had sent a short biography of himself that would be included in the program to be handed out to those attending, and Barbara, along with Vikki's assistant worked together to produce a flyer announcing the event that was distributed all over the cancer center and a couple of other high traffic areas around the University.

Barbara had occasionally made a casserole or a dessert to take to our monthly support group meetings, always receiving raves of appreciation, and so she thought with Mark, traveling down from Maryland to present the training program deserved lunch with more variety than the food we always received from The Biltmore Grille.

They generously donated lunch to us each month. The food that he prepared for the group was nutritious, easily swallowed and digested by cancer patients who were having trouble with their mouths and other issues. When she told Vikki about her idea, she thought it was a good one.

So Barbara, who loved to cook and experiment in the kitchen, began planning a menu for the event. Thinking it would be simple and not very expensive, at first we thought about paying for the meal ourselves. It quickly became obvious it would require more money than we could comfortably afford. Vikki suggested we save all of our receipts and she would ask the cancer center to reimburse us for the cost of the meal.

Barbara planned a great menu, all the while conscious that some people still had chewing and swallowing issues. She made sure to include things they would be able to enjoy as well.

Always a thrifty shopper who could buy groceries and other necessities and still be able to save money, Barbara sat down and first made a copy of the menu she would prepare. Then she made a list of the supplies she needed.

Instead of bulk shopping at one place, she spaced out the shopping. Whenever we were shopping, she would look for items she needed, and if they were on sale she bought them. Then she would circle them on the cash register receipt and put it aside to be turned into Diane Cole.

She shopped at Farmer Fresh in Louisa, the Dollar Tree in Charlottesville, The Dollar Store, Food Lion and Great Valu in Greene County and bought all of the fresh fruit and produce from Carl Ragland, who gave her a discount since it was for a cancer program.

The menu planned was a combination of tastes and textures people could choose from according to their likes, dislikes and their ability to eat. Whether the problem stemmed from dry mouth, chewing or swallowing difficulties, there was something for everyone.

There was Salmon Quiche which Barbara found in a book published by SPOHNC titled "We have Walked In Your Shoes", Garden Macaroni Salad (where she used fresh made Ranch Dressing instead of mayonnaise), Hot Beef and Pasta Salad, Potato, Ham & Broccoli Casserole, Lemon Pound Cake, Orange Pound Cake, Country Fruit Bread, Zucchini Bread, Banana Bread, assorted fruit juices and water.

To make some of the dishes more palatable for cancer patients she either substituted chopped varieties of the vegetables or meats, or using our electric chopper made her own.

The entire week before the meeting Barbara was in the kitchen, her apron on and all of her baking pans and utensils in constant use, as she worked on preparing the dishes. She had devised a schedule to have all of them done by early to mid morning on Thursday.

The hot foods would be the last ones she would prepare. She baked the breads and cakes, frosting, slicing and storing them in airtight containers to lock in freshness; she chopped vegetables for the salad, vegetables for the casseroles, chopped ham and grated cheese. In between each batch of bread, she cleaned bowls and utensils, and preparing the next batch as one baked. She also made a loaf of banana bread and country fruit bread for Mark to take back home with him.

The last dish to be made was the Salmon Quiche, which since she was making six of them, and they needed to be hot; she got up at 4 a.m., and had the first two in the oven by five O'clock.

At ten am, as I was carrying the dishes out to the car and loading them, she was on the telephone with Vikki for any last minute detail concerning the meeting. Vikki, having to go to Biltmore Grille to pick up the dishes they donated, asked if we would get there to welcome Mark in her place and she would be there as quickly as possible. Never having seen Mark except on the advocacy training video on NCCS' website, she assured Vikki that it wouldn't be a problem and that we would be glad to do it.

Little did either of us realize at that moment, but we were in for a surprise when he arrived.

When the date for the event (July 26, 2007) had been finalized, Vikki talked with the staff at the Forestry Building to obtain a bigger room than the one where we usually meet because we were expecting a fairly large turn-out, and they had given us the Executive Board Room upstairs on the second floor, where we would also have access to a kitchen area for heating food, keeping them chilled and enough counter space to setting it up buffet style.

Barbara and I took the elevator upstairs and checked out both areas before I began to unload the car. I would bring the food upstairs and she would set it out, or if needed, place it in the oven to reheat.

Mark had said that he would be arriving around 11ish, and when the time came and we hadn't seen him, Barbara began wondering what was keeping him.

Shortly after uttering those words, two gentlemen came up the stairs, walking into the Board Room and looking around. Barbara, who was sitting in one of the chairs in the "lobby" between the kitchen and board room, wondered if one of them was Mark, and asked me to go find out.

Uh huh, no way; I wasn't going to embarrass myself, so I told her to do it. Well, they kind of met right outside the room, with each repeating the others names and no introductions were needed after that. They hugged, and we all shook hands, and Mark introduced us to Dan Waeger who had accompanied him.

Barbara got a little embarrassed when she told Mark she didn't recognize him because he didn't look anything like he did in the training video on the website.

They unloaded their material and Barbara helped set up the room for the presentation before going back to finish the food preparation, and had just finished when Vikki, and Gordon arrived with the other food and plates and accessories.

The first part of the meeting concerned Second Wind, where everyone introduced themselves and told a little about their diagnosis, treatment and prognosis and then a couple of business items were dealt with quickly, and then my wife was totally shocked and rendered speechless by what happened.

Vikki, unknown to Barbara, had had a certificate of appreciation made up for her for all of the work that she had done to make the program possible and a success, and also presented her with a plant: a beautiful yellow Chrysanthemum on behalf of Second Wind.

Mark's Presentation in PowerPoint was informative and very well received by everyone in attendance. He included some of his experience with cancer: He is a 4 time survivor of melanoma and his last recurrence had occurred in January of 2005.

He began working with NCCS in late 2000, started as a volunteer and eventually moving into a staff position, and currently holds the title of Director of Survivorship Policy. Dan Waeger is Manager of Development with NCCS and is currently undergoing treatment after being diagnosed with double lung cancer, and at the time of the presentation, was disease free in one lung, and still receiving treatment on the other.

Dan's story was especially touching. He is in his early 20's, and has never been a smoker. However, he was diagnosed with double lung cancer, and has been through extensive treatments with chemotherapy and radiation therapy. One of his lungs has already healed, and the doctors, according to Dan, are very hopeful about his prognosis. His attitude: friendly, open, honest, caring and so positive, as he shared his story, was very inspirational and moving.

We were very glad that the program had been so well received and that it was a very successful venture. It made us feel good to have a part in bringing something useful to other patients and survivors and their families.

Behind the Scenes

Barbara became committed to researching and finding information about cancer.

She didn't limit herself to any one subject. All information about the different types of treatments, how to deal with the side effects, and what those side effects could include at the different stages, and anything else that she felt was important. She also looked for anything that would have any sort of impact on me personally or on our lives while I was going through my own stages. The more she learned, the more she researched.

I was so focused on just surviving the day-to-day events of treatments that it never occurred to me to seek out information from my doctors. Or that there was information available in each of the clinics I went to. I showed up for appointments and whatever test or other procedure they told me I needed. Beyond that, I didn't worry about it. I dealt with one thing at a time, and it still seemed to be coming at me like a run away freight train sometimes.

Barbara, on the other hand kept a daily journal of my symptoms, all of the drugs prescribed, any side effects I had, a list of my doctors and their contact information. She also had a growing list of all of the agencies she had contacted and what the results of those contacts were: whether she had or had not received help from them.

NCCS offers a variety of publications and materials designed as resources for patients and their families and one of the best resources is the audio compact disc set called the Cancer Survival Toolbox. She worked with Mark Gorman and brought multiple copies of the Toolbox, (which covers topics like Communicating, Finding Information, Making Decisions, Solving Problems, Negotiating, Standing Up for Your Rights, Topics for Older Persons, Finding Ways to Pay for Care, Caring for the Caregiver, Living Beyond Cancer) to the Cancer Center, the ENT Clinic, Radiology/Oncology and to our support group.

She also spent time on NCCS' website downloading the manuscripts that went along with each section and then printing them out making three copies and putting them into a manual for patients who would prefer to have the information in written form. One manual was given to each of the areas that had the audio discs.

She has written to the Lance Armstrong Foundation and received multiple copies of his Survivor Notebook for individual patients as well as for the social workers in the Cancer Center, and has ordered cases of information booklets from the Foundation for our group as well as the ENT Clinic, always keeping extra in case she runs across someone personally who needs information and doesn't know where to turn.

She has ordered samples of products from several Pharmaceutical companies to share with our group and other cancer patients and is always searching for reliable information for her resource database that she willingly shares with others.

In January of 2008, she assumed the responsibility of writing our support group's monthly newsletter when the former editor decided to cut back on the amount of volunteer projects he had, and she is always looking for information to share that will make a difference.

When I was a patient in the cancer center receiving Chemotherapy, one thing that I found meant a lot to me was that there were snack foods: fruit, snack cakes, brownies or cookies that were offered to us as we sat in those chairs for hours on end.

It often soothed frazzled nerves, calmed upset stomachs or quieted the hunger pangs we were experiencing.

At least once a month, my wife takes time out to spend a day in the kitchen baking different breads, pound cakes, cookies or brownies which she takes into the patients as her way of saying thank you for all they did for me.

It makes us both feel so good when the staff smiles and appreciates what we do, or a patient says thank you with a smile or a touch, or asks Barbara for the recipe because they enjoyed it so much.

I think it should be duly noted that the caring and compassionate attitude of the nursing staff in the Infusion and the Radiation Clinics, along with the nursing staff and the technicians, helped me get through the long and often stressful days of treatment.

Their bright smiles and friendly attitude helped me overcome some of the depression that is often normal and expected when dealing with chronic and debilitating diseases.

Barbara was instrumental in getting me to share with these staff members some of my problems and concerns. She would call and ask any question, not caring if it sounded stupid or not if it was something that she wanted to find out about.

I guess it eventually rubbed off on me and I started following in her footsteps. Whoever said you can't teach an old dog a new trick?

Barbara has also taken on the responsibility of becoming a full voting member of C-PAC—Cancer Project Action Committee, as part of the Commonwealth of Virginia's State Cancer Plan

We attended a quarterly meeting of the Committee held in the Jordan Hall Auditorium at the University of Virginia on November 13, 2007. Diane Cole, along with Carole Havrila gave the address concerning Integrative Medicine and the importance of good nutrition, respectively.

At the end of the meeting, Barbara asked to be assigned to the Survivorship Committee which will coincide with her work with Mark Gorman and NCCS.

Barbara wanted to share with people how cancer can impact and change a person's life forever—how no part of it is untouched by the devastating disease. She started out to just write a short, simple little "paper" she could share with our group and maybe a few close friends.

But as she began typing, she realized that, perhaps—just maybe, some of the things that I had gone through: accepting the diagnosis, dealing with the various government agencies, peoples attitudes, struggling with bills and creditors, wondering how one loss after the other would affect my quality of life—maybe all of it could help others who would be coming behind me, and would be traveling on this long and often endless road.

While there are a lot of negative things we deal with—there are often blessings and rays of sunshine, miracles and generosity in places we least expect them. So, she sat down, and painstakingly went back over notes and memories to put together this book to bring hope to those feeling hopeless, and to bring awareness to the fact that we are cancer patients, but most importantly we are SURVIVORS!!!

INDEPENDENT AGAIN!

When I was diagnosed with cancer I didn't want to be a burden on anyone, and I certainly had no intention of becoming a charity case. I didn't want to have to sit around waiting for someone to give me the necessities and other things that I felt I needed in order to survive. It irked the hell out of me to me totally dependent on "Uncle Sam" each month, when I received my disability check. Now wait a minute, don't get me wrong. I think that disability can be a good thing—I am all for it.

It just wasn't for me. I wanted to work. I had been working at one job or another since I was in high school, and certainly since graduating. I admit I job hopped for a lot of my work history, but I still worked. I didn't rely on anybody else. Receiving the disability now, in what should have been the prime of my life made me feel degraded, angry, very frustrated and useless.

It wasn't all just about how I felt. Social Security Disability isn't intended for people who have a lot of expenses every month. Barbara and I barely scraped by and it was so damn hard to be forced to choose which bill would get paid when. It was like robbing Peter to pay Paul.

There were times when I wanted to call Social Security and tell them to keep the damn check. That I was barely surviving on the amount I was getting and that I was going to suck it up and go back to work. But thank God, common sense would kick back in just in time to keep me from making a complete fool out of myself.

Mentally and emotionally I rebelled at being held back. But physically I was still going through so much there was nothing I could do but to keep relying on the government. I began to understand why they have the five-year watch program for cancer patients.

I knew that I couldn't go to work without the approval of Dr. Reibel, so I decided to discuss it with him when I saw him for my scheduled checkup. He didn't say I could or couldn't go to work, but that it was up to me and how I felt about it, but that if a prospective employer needed anything from him to just fax him the paperwork and he would fill it out for me. Hallelujah! At least I could count on him to back up any decision I made.

As anxious as I was to go back to work, I knew I couldn't jeopardize the disability, and before I could make any informed decision I needed more information. How would working affect my payment? How many hours could I work? Was there a limit on the amount I could earn? How long would it be before my checks would be stopped?

I paid a visit to our local Social Security office in Charlottesville VA to find out the answers. I found out there was what they call a trial work period in the fine print of disability, so that a person receiving disability to work full time up to nine months without interruption of their benefits.

There was no limit on the amount you could earn within those nine months, because it was to see if you could become gainfully employed again. Well, now I thought—there could be a silver lining here after all.

I was still experiencing spasms in my throat that were painful and would cause me to clutch at my throat with my hand and breathe harshly or sometimes to even hold my breath until after it passed, and there is still some joint stiffness in my shoulder and it ached, but I had learned to accept. Dr. Read had prescribed Pentoxifylline, 400 mg twice a day and when it didn't control it very well, he increased it to three times a day.

Whatever job I decided to take it would have to be something that while active, was not too strenuous. I could not put undue pressure on my neck and shoulder.

One of the jobs I had held in the past that I was both good at and enjoyed for the most part, had been as a Housekeeper Technician II in the Operating Room (how ironic) at UVa.

It had been when ServiceMaster had control of the contract for cleaning the hospital and all of the outbuildings. I didn't know if there were any job openings there, but figured it was as good a place to start looking as any.

A new company out of Wayne, Pennsylvania—Crothall Healthcare, Incorporated had won the bid as the new contractor for UVa, so I needed to go to the Environmental Services Department, located on zero level, to find out if there were any job openings available for a housekeeper.

I went in and picked up the application because I wanted to bring it home so that Barbara could help me fill it out. I still have problems writing for extended periods of time due to arthritis and carpal tunnel syndrome.

One of the other side effects from chemotherapy was what medical scientists now call Chemo Brain. It affects your thinking ability, your attention span and you have difficulty hearing and comprehending at times. It isn't too bad in my particular case, just enough to be annoying.

After finishing the application, I returned it to the office and was told someone would be in touch with me later. I waited for about a week and telephoned them. I was never able to talk to the person I was referred to and after several calls, was finally told to come in for an interview. All things considered the interview went well.

My next thing was to see my doctor for a letter of release to return to work, because I was a cancer patient, whether I was in survivorship stage or not. Ellen Desper wrote the letter for me and when I turned it in, I was scheduled for an orientation.

The orientation is rather boring because they go over a lot things that are just common sense, but it is mandatory, so we all had to suffer through it. The supervisor who was conducting the orientation didn't show up for work the second day we were scheduled, and we were assigned to work on the floors with a housekeeper who had been working there for a while.

On my first day I encountered a problem with one of the supervisors over my water bottle. She said I couldn't have it on the floor with me because it was a safety risk and that it was against the rules and regulations. She told me I would have to drink from the water cooler like everyone else.

I have problems drinking from any container without the aid of a straw. Although I tried to explain to her I had to have it because I suffered from dry mouth due to radiation treatment, she wouldn't budge. Barbara called the ENT clinic the following day and it was taken care of by Ellen Desper.

I was ecstatic and ready to walk on air that I was gainfully employed one more time. It made me feel useful again, like I had some semblance of control over part of my life. Mentally I felt relief, maybe it wouldn't be so hard on either Barbara or me anymore—struggling, depressed and worried constantly, and I had something to look forward to each and every day.

I was able to get out of the confines of the house and those walls that lurked dangerously close as if to suffocate me. Of course, going back to work now, after battling cancer and the treatments wasn't as easy as it had been before.

There were a lot of things I had to compensate for and work around to make it suitable for me. I was still having problems gaining weight no matter what and how often I ate. I had to remember to pack nutritious snacks and a balanced dinner, along with plenty of liquids for hydration and Ensure for energy. Larry Haywood had suggested in one of our group meetings to substitute at least one Gatorade for a bottle of water per day, in order to keep our electrolytes balanced.

I took quick little breaks several times a day, including my regularly scheduled ones, which helped a lot. By the time I got home though, I was literally exhausted. Sometimes, I would sit up and have something to drink and Barbara and I would talk for a while so I could relax and chill out before going to bed.

Well, we can't expect it to be perfect, right? The one drawback, for me—was I would be working second shift—3 pm until midnight. All of my other jobs had always been during first shift, normal business hours, so this was a major adjustment for me.

I was used to eating dinner at a normal hour and relaxing in front of the television. I was usually well into my second dream by the time I would be getting off from work. There was the question of how much rest I would get.

I have never been a person who could sleep during the day even when I was sick. The sunlight outside was too tempting. Being able to do chores around the house and resting would take a lot of getting used to. Barbara would have a period of adjustment as well. For me it was having time during the day to do odd jobs like cutting the grass; and for her, it was when to prepare breakfast and dinner. When would we take care of personal business or doctor appointments?

There were also the support group meetings—which were still a key part of my survivorship. They were something we didn't want to miss. They always seemed to be on the Thursday I was scheduled to work. Thankfully, my supervisors were willing to let me switch my days off for important events dealing with my cancer so I wouldn't miss any of it.

The way the Crothall staff did things as far as office work, making sure that the workers had the proper equipment and supplies to work with, or to have help from a supervisor when it was needed left a lot to be desired and oftentimes, was non-existent to the point of being exasperating.

For example, the supervisor that I was assigned either had the day or was on vacation more than she worked, or would call over to my job site saying that she was coming over there and then would never show up.

When it came to having the proper supplies, forget about it! A lot of times I would have to use my own personal car and load it down with as much of the materials that I could stuff into it and then take time away from when I was supposed to be cleaning or doing the trash and bio-hazard pulls to unload and stock the supply closet. And of course, there were just the little things that would irritate the hell out of somebody that should never have occurred.

I tried often to overlook it but I am afraid that there were a lot of times when I got home that Barbara literally had to yell at me to leave the job at the job or I would have driven her stark raving mad because of the things I kept complaining about.!

Most of the people who worked in the CORE Lab where I was assigned were really nice and friendly and we all got along great. I made a lot of good friends among the staff and with my work ethics and attention to detail I earned a lot of respect from them.

When I was eventually forced to switch to part-time before the end of my nine months in order to keep my disability payments, they all missed me because most of the work during the day was being neglected or just haphazardly done.

Barbara made a great big impression on them too during the Christmas holiday when she presented the staff with a tray of homemade goodies for them to enjoy and a card for them from the both of us.

I eventually left the job altogether on January 8, 2008, in order to take a better paying job and it had much more desirable hours since it was during the day. It wasn't what I wanted, but hey at $10.00 an hour and only having to work for 5 hours a day, who could complain too much.

It was still cleaning, but not the same type of thorough cleaning I was accustomed to doing in the CORE Lab. This was janitorial cleaning at the UPS Building in Charlottesville.

I had found the job advertised in our local paper, and called and left my name and phone number on an answering machine, wondering if anyone would call me back.

A couple of days later, the owner of the company, Allied Janitorial Services in Madison Heights, VA called me. He was very up-front and had a good attitude on the telephone. His name was Frank West, and he said that he had been doing this type of work for 35 years. I was amazed.

He was looking for someone to work part time, which fit right into what I wanted because of my disability.

I explained to him that I had gone through cancer and all of the treatments and that I was still on disability but working for Crothall, and needed part-time work to keep my checks. He asked me to go by the UPS building and check it out and let him know if I still wanted it.

When Barbara went to her doctor appointment I went up there to meet Eric, his son. It really did seem like a good job for me and something that I would be comfortable with. His son said that he had a couple of more people to interview but that he would tell his dad that he was impressed with the way I handled myself during the interview and that he would call me later that afternoon.

When I didn't hear anything from him, I called the number in the paper and spoke with his dad again, and confirmed that I did want the job. He called me back less than an hour later and asked me when I could start!

Tired of working the nights and now every weekend, I answered quickly that I could start the next day. He told me to be at the shop as they call UPS by 7 a.m.

Looking back now, I realize that perhaps I moved a little too hastily in quitting the job I was good at and was for the most part comfortable with. But that's exactly what I did.

I called into the office at Crothall and told them that I had taken another job and that I wouldn't be coming back, since I was scheduled to work that weekend. I did want to give them the chance to find someone to take my place, after all—and not leave them with nobody there.

Well it seemed like it wasn't such a good idea the second day at UPS. Eric, the owner's son didn't seem to appreciate that I move a little slower than most people but do get everything done. Besides, I felt like I needed the chance to familiarize myself with the set up and operation that they had there since it was a lot different than what I was used to.

Well, thankfully they are still letting me work, but it's frustrating because when I go in each morning, I can't help but wonder if this will be the day that he tells me he can't use me anymore. Maybe I should have kept the other one?

Only time will tell…

FROM PATIENT TO ADVOCATE

The National Coalition for Cancer Survivorship is the sponsor of a bill, H.R. 1078—The Comprehensive Cancer Care Improvement Act, that would provide quality care for all cancer patients and survivors, and they had been working with members of the U.S. House of Representatives in order to get members to sign on in support of the bill.

Barbara and I were both excited about working with Mark to ensure that the bill would be passed. It has so many things that patients, their care givers and others who work with them throughout their treatment could benefit from. For Barbara and I, the key advantages the plan offered were:

By establishing a cancer care plan at the start of treatments it would allow the patient to be more involved in their treatments and they will know about and be able to understand each phase, which will make them feel more comfortable and less stressed. They will also be able to chart their progress, along with their physician.

The transition from "patient" to "survivor" is a difficult one for patients to cope with. Other than regularly scheduled "maintenance" checks by their radiologist/oncologist or their surgeon, they often feel abandoned. At the present time, patients are left on their own when it comes to dealing with any kind of follow-up care for pain management and other medical issues. These most often arise after the completion of treatment. The advantage of having a written follow-up plan is that they can refer to it to see what tests and or treatments they might need, and the feeling of being "lost" or "forgotten" will be alleviated as they continue in their recovery.

Symptom management, along with the Comprehensive Care plan is very much needed by all cancer patients and survivors. A diagnosis of cancer changes a person's life forever and there is no "speedy recovery." They cope with side effects and limitations for the rest of their lives. By training their healthcare professionals, the professionals will be able to recognize and treat the patient effectively and efficiently, which will reassure the patient that they are receiving the best cancer care available. With this being incorporated into their existing cancer care plan, it is a cost-effective measure that prevents other expensive or long-term treatments in the future by addressing the problem as it occurs.

Barbara began working with Mark on this part of the advocacy, and since she had worked with Congressman Virgil H. Goode, Jr. (5th District Representative) in the past on several personal issues, (Republican Pig Roasts in Greene County, and help in obtaining her Social Security Disability), she volunteered to speak with him in order to obtain his signature of support.

When he was in Charlottesville to present the cancer advocacy program, Mark had brought copies of the Commonwealth's Representatives with him as a handout, along with congressional district maps and a copy of his presentation.

Barbara, using the handout, called Congressman Goode's Charlottesville office to ask for an appointment, and his office manager informed her that he had held appointments there a week ago, and he was now in his Rocky Mount, Virginia office (which is also where he and his family live). She directed Barbara to the Congressman's appointment secretary in his Danville, Virginia office.

When she called to request the interview, the Congressman's appointment secretary asked her to send the Congressman a handwritten letter explaining why she wanted a meeting with him and he would respond either granting or denying her the meeting.

She gave her the address of his Rocky Mount, Virginia office, where she suggested Barbara mail the letter. Several days later, she received a written response from Congressman Goode, before she'd ever had time to write to him.

He thanked her for contacting his office, and stating that she could call to schedule an appointment with his D.C. office before October, or to call his district office in Charlottesville after October 10th to schedule a meeting on his next day there.

Barbara, wanting to discuss the options with Mark before making a commitment, telephoned him at NCCS, only to discover that he was out of the office on vacation for a couple of days.

Early the following morning as we were having coffee, the telephone rang and it was Congressman Goode's appointment secretary calling. She said the Congressman had an appointment opening in his Washington, D.C. office on August 6, 2007, and would like to know if we could be there by 11 a.m.

My wife was shocked by the invitation being issued, but after checking the calendar to see if I was off from work, she quickly confirmed that we would be there.

When Barbara was finally able to get in touch with Mark and informed him of the things she had accomplished since their last telephone conversation, he was delighted to learn about it, and was willing to help her prepare a presentation packet to deliver to the Congressman when we met with him.

He mailed her several copies of the overview for H.R. 1078, a copy of a letter of support from the Massey Cancer Center in Richmond, VA (only one of two NCI Designated Cancer Centers in Virginia), and a copy of all the organizations who were supporting the legislation.

He suggested that we get a letter of support from the cancer center at the University of Virginia to include in the presentation. That would be a problem.

It was not because the cancer center wasn't in support of the bill, everyone there was. However, because the University of Virginia is a state funded institution they were not legally able to write a letter to support any political stands on issues, or they would risk losing their funding. However, all was not lost as far as letters of support.

Through persistence and determination, Diane Cole and Vikki Bravo wrote a letter supporting the legislation, and all members of the support staff (chaplain, dietician, navigator, manager, social workers) all signed it.

Barbara was also able to get letters from Ellen Desper, R.N. in the ENT Clinic and from Dr. Paul Read, Associate Professor of Radiology/Oncology, to add to her arsenal.

This would be our first trip to Capitol Hill, and we were at loss on where to go or how to find our way around, and Mark, understanding this, volunteered to be our navigator for the day.

We were really excited about going, and it would be good to see Mark again, and be able to work on such an important issue. However, Barbara wasn't finished with her work for the trip. She was trying to accomplish as much as she could with the opportunity that she had been given.

When the appointment with Congressman Goode had been made and confirmed with another telephone call, Barbara once again gathered her materials and contacted the office of Congressman Eric I. Cantor (6th District Representative), who was actually our representative for our location, and asked if it would be possible to speak with one of his Legislative Assistants on Healthcare.

The first time she called, she got the brush off, which didn't deter her. She called back within the hour, and this time her call was transferred to his Washington office.

She spoke with Miss. Lindsay Shore in his office, and discovering that she was his healthcare assistant, explained she wanted the chance to meet and discuss the importance of the Cancer Care Improvement Act to cancer patients, survivors and their families.

She told Miss Shore we had an appointment scheduled in Congressman Goode's office, and asked if she could meet with her after that. Miss Shore scheduled the appointment for one O'clock the same afternoon.

Congressman Robert "Bob" Goodlatte (6th District Representative) was the only other member of the Virginia Delegation within driving distance of our home who had not yet signed on in support of the legislation.

When Barbara telephoned his Harrisonburg Virginia office she received a brisk brush off several times. Finally, she was directed by his District Representative to contact Jessica Orsulak, his appointment setter in his D.C. office to schedule an appointment.

It was several days later when she finally got the call that they would be glad to schedule an appointment for us to see one of his assistants on August 6th while we were in Washington.

We both wanted to make a good impression since it was Capitol Hill, and we were meeting with Congressmen or their associates and we spent time before the trip for both of us to visit the hair salon and barber shop, respectively.

We then went through our closets to choose appropriate clothing, and deciding that my suit and ties were ok, Barbara didn't like what she had available, so it was off to Wal-Mart to buy a new outfit.

She wanted something that was easy care and color coordinated, but cool and comfortable since she would be sitting in her manual wheelchair a lot that day as we traveled from one location to the other.

She finally chose a pair of chocolate brown cotton dress slacks with a multi colored brown print leopard pull over dress t-shirt, a pair of white canvas slip on shoes and a coordinated white handbag, and completed the ensemble with a pair of gold hoop earrings and a gold dress watch. I was surprised by her thriftiness as the entire purchase price was $50.

I wore a blue tie, white dress shirt and blue pants from one of my suits, along with my black dress shoes. I decided since the weather was hot I wouldn't need the jacket to the suit.

We set our alarm for five O'clock the morning of the 6th in order to have time to shower, dress and enjoy a cup of coffee before setting out on the trip. We were planning on stopping at McDonald's in Madison, since it was on the way and have breakfast, because if I don't eat I get nervous, shaky and weak.

As we were just coming onto Route 66, Mark called Barbara on her cellular phone (it's a Trac Fone where you buy minutes), and she told him that we'd be in Vienna in about an hour. He was still in Silver Spring and planning to leave the office to take the Metro into the Capitol south and would be in D.C. about 10:30.

The traffic was heavy and fast on Route 66, and the exit lanes can be quite confusing if you aren't paying close attention, because some of the lanes turn into exit lanes without warning, and you have to get over into another lane to prevent getting off before you want or are supposed to.

Mark had emailed Barbara the directions to the Metro station in Vienna, and when we got there and moved onto the parking deck, there were no spaces available. After riding it twice, we had no choice except to park behind a truck pulled over to the side, next to one of the concrete walls and walk for a good distance.

It was a little hard pushing the manual chair but we managed to make it to the station, and then had to ask directions on where to go since we weren't familiar with how the system worked.

One of the attendants inside where you purchase the tickets was kind enough to help us and to tell us which train we needed to board on the loading platform, and we had to take an elevator down to it.

Barbara called Mark on her cellular phone to let him know that we were on the Metro heading into the City, and because we didn't have a schedule with the names of the stops along the way, Mark told her which one to look for so that we knew Metro South was the next stop and that he would be waiting for us inside the station.

When we got there, Mark was actually on the platform as the doors opened and helped me push Barbara's chair off and onto the platform.

From there we left the Metro station to walk the few blocks to the Longworth House Office Building, where Congressman Goode's office is located. The brick sidewalks of Washington are in sad need of repair, with a lot of the bricks loose and standing at angles that make it very tricky to walk or traverse with a wheelchair, often causing a person to trip or the chair to bump along.

As we were making our way to "the hill" as people there refer to it, Barbara was busy looking around at the different buildings, massive in size and in "rows", one after the other, as she kept up a running dialogue with Mark who sometimes walked ahead of us and sometimes behind us. He was there to take the lead, for which we were thankful—because I'd have been at a total loss where to go.

We located the handicapped entrance and entered the building. Security guards were stationed there and greeted us warmly. We put our bags and cellular phones on the conveyor, and then Mark and I walked through the sensors while the lady ran a wand over Barbara as she sat in her chair, and we were cleared for entrance, and the day began.

Before we approached Congressman Goode's office, we located restrooms and each of us took turns, and freshened up before we went into the meeting.

It was impressive going down the halls, with "suites" that held the Congressmen's offices lined up on each side, and a Bronze plate mounted on the wall beside each entrance that held the Congressman's name, state he represented, and there was an "official" flag and the American flag on each side of the door.

When we were ready to enter the suite, I said to my wife I wasn't sure if I could do this or not. I have a speech impediment and I am very self-conscious about it. I never know when it will flare up, but often times it is when I am nervous or unsure of myself.

She told me not to worry about it, that I would be fine because he was a man just like me and put his pants on the same way I did, one leg at a time and that he worked for us and to just be myself.

When we walked into the suite, and gave our names to one of his staff members, we were asked to have a seat because he was on a telephone call and it would be a few minutes.

Barbara was glancing around the waiting area, and I could see the wheels turning inside her head as she took mental notes of the furnishings and everything else to be able to describe it in detail to our group and all of the people who knew we were on this trip today.

Looking around myself, I was impressed. Matt Bravo, (as his name plate on his desk identified him) was very open and friendly when we had entered, and greeted us very warmly and courteously.

It turned out that Matt is one of Congressman Goode's Legislative Assistants, and since that first time in his office, he and Barbara have had a few other telephone conversations.

The waiting area was carpeted in deep rich blue carpet, very thick and the furnishings were cherry, and the cushions on the chairs and sofas matched the carpeting, except it had small yellow designs on mixed in.

Mark had chosen to stay outside in the hallway and watch over the wheelchair and Barbara's briefcase since he said that we were the advocates and he was just our navigator.

Yes, he was showing us around and where to go for the day, but just a navigator doesn't do credit to what he was for us.

If it hadn't been for Mark and NCCS then we'd never have been in Washington, or for that matter, we'd never have known that we could request meetings with Congressmen and that what we had to say about legislation would matter to them.

Several minutes later, we were told to go on into his office by the staff member.

As we entered the inner office, Congressman Goode stood up and came around his desk, welcoming us inside and asked us to have a seat after shaking hands with us both. Barbara seemed totally relaxed and at ease, while I was nervous and a little unsure of myself.

The office was large and comfortable, with seating spaced out in an informal setting. The Congressman's desk was a large deep rich cherry, with lots of family photos displayed along with his computer and telephone, and a well maintained calendar and writing pad. There were floor-to-ceiling bookcases that housed leather bound books, most of which were law books, and a few potted plants placed strategically to absorb sunlight filtering through the window.

The first thing he did after having a seat back in his chair was to ask about how our trip up to D.C. had gone, and then we talked a little about the upcoming Republican Pig Roast scheduled for sometime in October, in Stanardsville, VA. Barbara used to attend them every year, especially when helping friends she knew campaign for local offices, so she and the Congressman had that in common and they discussed it for a few minutes.

I was beginning to feel more at ease, because it felt as if we were sitting in our living room or kitchen talking instead of in the Capitol.

He asked me questions about my cancer: the type I'd been diagnosed with, the treatments I'd taken, and what side effects I'd had to deal with and then we talked about our support group before the purpose of our meeting ever came up.

Barbara answered all of the questions that he asked, and told how she thought that it would help patients, their caregivers and their families. She gave him the information packet that we had put together, and he took it and said that he was looking forward to reading it and in getting the report back from the committee.

He was very up front about being in support of the bill but would like to wait until the report came in before signing onto it As we prepared to leave, we asked if we could have our picture taken with him, and we took it outside of the office in the hallway with the flags on each side of us.

After we left Congressman Goode's office, Mark suggested we grab some lunch before going to meet with Lindsay Shore in Eric Cantor's office. It sounded like a good plan to me. I was a little hungry and the water in my bottle had gotten warm and wasn't very refreshing at this point. With all of the walking that we had already done, plus pushing the manual wheelchair, I had long since worked off the breakfast we had at McDonald's.

Mark took us to the cafeteria in the Cannon House Building, which was a little busy. Barbara and I ordered a hamburger with lettuce, tomato, mayonnaise and onions and an order of French fries. The fries were different than what we were used to, and were served in a paper cup. Barbara decided to stay in her chair and Mark helped her with a tray so she could hold everything.

After lunch, it was off to the meeting with Lindsay Shore.

As we made our way down the many corridors between the three buildings which are home to the U.S. House of Representatives, we found pictures displayed that showed the actual construction of one of the buildings, from the conception and breaking ground, through each stage of construction to the completion and we took several minutes to examine each one, finding it very interesting.

When we got to the office, she was waiting for our arrival. Barbara had talked to her several times on the telephone and she was surprised to find that Lindsay was younger than she had anticipated.

She was very friendly and forthcoming in her greeting, shaking hands with both of us enthusiastically as she invited us into the conference room.

After we were seated, she asked about our drive into the city and we chit chatted for a bit. Then she stated what we were there to discuss, rather than ask it as a question. She had taken time to read over the Bill before we got there, and was really excited about what she had learned.

She thought Congressman Cantor would have no problem in offering his support for the legislation.

She was open and candid throughout the meeting, and shared personal experiences she and her family had gone through with cancer, and so she was well aware of how debilitating the disease is and how it wreaks havoc in a person's life.

She went to her computer and tracked the bill to see which committee had it on their schedule at that time. It is in the House Ways and Means Committee, one of the committees on which Congressman Cantor is a member.

She promised to keep in touch with any new developments, and before we knew it; we had actually spent close to 2 hours in the meeting.

When we walked out into the reception area, it was good to see that Mark had decided to come inside and make himself comfortable. He and Lindsay shook hands and we all chatted for a few minutes before we left to head over to our next meeting, with Congressman Goodlatte's office.

The Rayburn House Office Building is the largest of the three buildings containing the U.S. House of Representatives. It took a while for us to make our way to Congressman Goodlatte's office, which was located at the back of the building.

When we walked into the office, we knew that this meeting was not going to go as smoothly or be as successful as the other two had been. The receptionist didn't seem to know who we were supposed to be meeting with, and we were forced to wait for several minutes.

During that time, the receptionist was trying to find the person who had granted our meeting; Barbara took the time to gather some of the business cards from the display on the counter, to add to her growing collection.

We were shown into a small conference room and were joined shortly by Kathryn Rexrode, who it turned out, was the Communications Director and Legislative Assistant to the Congressman. We were very disappointed from the very onset of the meeting.

Unlike with Virgil Goode and Lindsay Shore, Miss Rexrode didn't seem to have any idea why we had requested the meeting. Barbara had been very specific on the telephone when she had called. We could tell that she wasn't very interested in what we were saying.

She went off on a new subject, talking about the area of Virginia where we live, and how much she and her husband enjoyed driving through on their way to the Harrisonburg District Office.

When we met Mark outside, she handed him the business cards and we made our way back to where we had originally entered the Longworth House Office Building. The heat, so humid you could have cut it with a knife, hit us full force as we stepped outside the building, causing us to gasp from the intensity.

We made our way back to the Metro station, only to discover the elevator leading down to the train was out of order. Mark offered to call a cab by using his cell phone, but one of the women who worked at the station said that she would have someone call a shuttle to take us to the next station, instead.

We had to wait for about half an hour before it arrived. We were able to get on the train and head back to Vienna. Mark rode with us to his stop, shaking my hand and giving Barbara a hug before disembarking.

He had been gracious enough to lend us his Metro pass, which would save money at the parking deck when we arrived back in Vienna. Barbara had promised to send it back in the mail the following day.

The Metro became more and more crowded since it was the end of the day, and people were on their way home from work or other business they'd done for the day. The perfumes and colognes had Barbara's asthma kicking up big time by the time we finally got off.

We were both parched and desperately wanting something cool to drink, and there wasn't a vending machine in sight! We did finally locate a bathroom and water cooler—which we drank from for a long time, before we made our way out of the station.

Barbara used her cell phone to call Vikki and let her know that we were safely back in Virginia, and should be home in a couple of hours, and promised to call her the following day to fill her in on all of the details of the trip.

We got home around seven O'clock that night, after stopping for a bite to eat, something cool to drink and to use the restroom at a local McDonald's on the way.

My feet were aching and tired from wearing my suede boots and all I wanted was to get into my pajamas and relax. Pushing her manual chair had been a chore, and one I didn't want to repeat any time soon!

LENDER, LENDER!

Barbara had tried unsuccessfully for over a year to obtain a scooter that would give her greater mobility without having to depend on me each and every time she wanted to go somewhere. The manual chair, while it allowed her to shop in places that didn't have Mart-Carts, or that were too large for her to shop walking short distances, meant that she needed help moving it around.

She could wheel it for short distances, but would often become winded. It would bring on severe coughing attacks that usually ended when she vomited, and her blood pressure had become elevated to the point her face was splotchy with red patches. So normally, we just shopped at Food Lion for groceries or at Wal-Mart for household supplies, unless I went to the other stores with list in hand.

I admit that Barbara had become so wrapped up in taking care of me and all of the stuff that it involved, and with the things she enjoyed doing for the cancer center and support group, that she had neglected several issues concerning her own health.

It wasn't that she intentionally did it. She relied on me for transportation and when I was on the restriction, it was hard to have means to do things like get groceries or for me to go to appointments— she refused to add anything else to the complicated maze.

Now, she finally started scheduling and keeping some of her doctor appointments, and one of the first she made was with her Primary Care

Physician, Dr. Michael Harper in the Family Medicine Clinic at the Primary Care Center at UVa. She wasn't particularly fond of him because they couldn't seem to get on the same page about some of the things she needed, so she never looked forward to the appointments.

She called and talked to several different representatives at the Scooter Store about how to get a scooter because of her limited mobility. When they did her application and verified her source and amount of income, she was eligible to receive it at little or reduced-cost. However, there was one major glitch. It involved Medicare, which will give you a hint that it was going to be a major headache to work out. They've never been known to be very cooperative or to do anything in a timely manner.

The Scooter Store couldn't process her application for the scooter because there was a red flag attached to her Medicare dating back to 1999. She had been involved in a motor vehicle accident that totaled her car, and she had to hire an attorney to handle the case.

Tom McGrath was an attorney in Richmond, Virginia who worked with motorcyclists, and she called him because he had worked with members of the outreach ministry at our church. He eventually settled the claim out of court and received his fee from the money paid to Barbara by the defendant.

For some reason, Medicare red flagged her file so any medical problems that arose at a later time, they assumed the defendant would be responsible for. It took almost three full months, a lot of telephone calls between my wife, the Scooter Store and Medicare before the issue was finally resolved to her satisfaction.

When she and the Scooter Store worked together, she discovered that living in a mobile home meant that a scooter was not the best option for her. They recommended a power chair instead. By this point, Barbara didn't really care as long as it was one or the other.

The next step involved Dr. Harper. They needed a prescription from him, stating it was a medically necessary piece of equipment before Medicare would pay the claim, minus the co-pay Barbara herself would be responsible for.

She was very skeptical about whether or not he would agree to write the prescription. But sheer determination kicked in, and she wasn't about to take no for an answer! When she went to the appointment, the last thing she said was that she would come out with the prescription. I had an appointment myself that day, and after taking her into the clinic, I had to leave.

She was in the exam room when Dr. Harper walked in and she swears to this day it was an imposter! He was very friendly, and this time he actually listened to what she had to say and didn't argue or interrupt her. And what really shocked her? He actually agreed that a scooter or power chair was what she needed to be able to get around independently.

He said that he would be glad to fill out all of the papers if they would just resend them. Evidently, when they had made the appointment and faxed them the first time, they had gotten misplaced and he had never received them.

Barbara asked him what he had done with the real Dr. Harper and he burst out laughing. He said he had finally decided to listen to patients first because he had gotten tired of being cursed out every day. He even wheeled her back into the waiting room himself when all of the nurses were busy with other patients.

Now that we knew she would be getting the power chair, we had another hurdle that we needed to overcome. How were we going to transport it? The only thing Medicare would pay for was the chair itself. They didn't help with ramps for taking the chair in and out of the home, or for lifts or carriers for an automobile to transport it. That would be up to us. Where to turn? Barbara began researching on the internet and in the telephone book for resources.

We had recently been working on getting a better car than the Ford Taurus, and had gone from a Dodge Stratus we had bought at The Auto Superstore in Charlottesville to a 2007 Kia Optima we bought with Price Kia right down the street from them on Pantops Mountain.

When Barbara finally located some places that had the lifts that were attached to the back bumpers of cars, she discovered they wouldn't work on our car. The Kia had bumpers which wouldn't support that amount of weight without bending, or if the bumper didn't bend the frame underneath would.

We thought about having a hitch attached and buying a small trailer, only to discover the price of those were way out of range for us, because none of the places offered a payment plan for people on limited income. So now what were we supposed to do?

At the time Barbara was going to a Chiropractor in Mechanicsville, Virginia in the hope that the therapy he offered would relieve some of the pressure and pain in her lower back.

One day when we left the appointment and stopped at a gas station, she looked up the address and telephone number of Congressman Eric Cantor's District Office in Glen Allen, and you wouldn't believe what she did next!

She had me drive down there, and she went in and talked with his District Representative, and actually told him she had a power chair and she needed help finding transportation to be able to haul it, and he even agreed to look into it for her!

When she finally became so exasperated she couldn't take anymore, Barbara decided to call the Department of Rehabilitative Services, with whom she had worked closely when she had been a student at Woodrow Wilson Rehabilitation Center years before.

She was hoping they had a program that would be helpful, or perhaps they would be able to point her in the right direction. After leaving a message with the Culpeper office that handled our locality, she finally received a call back a couple of days later.

The counselor she spoke with said the only program she knew to recommend was a low interest loan program called the Assistive Technology Loan Fund Authority. Barbara asked for their number, figuring it wouldn't hurt to look into it at this point.

She called and spoke one of the ladies in the office, who explained to her how the program worked. It was low-interest government loan for people with disabilities, and who needed help with transportation and other devices to be independent.

She asked a lot of questions to determine if we would be eligible for the program, and then for our mailing address so she could mail out the application we needed to complete and send back.

Once we did that, she ran all of the paperwork through their system to print out the necessary papers for the contract which she sent out to us. We needed to sign them in front of a Notary Public, and mail them back to her by the deadline.

In the meantime, since the loan would pay for a vehicle as well as the installation of a lift, we had to find both. The woman recommended Independent Lifestyles in Madison Heights for the lift, and Barbara had constantly been in touch with one of the specialists, Josh. She called and told him he needed to fax to LTFA the amount the lift was going to cost to purchase and install, which he did.

We had found a 2000 Dodge Grand Caravan in one of the papers in Richmond, that was similar in it's layout to the Blue Ridge Buck Saver from our days of doing the yard sales. It was located in Mechanicsville, not far from the Chiropractor Barbara was going to.

The guy was really nice and he had also faxed his information to ATLFA. We went to Bank of America, since we have a checking account there, and had the papers notarized and sent them out the same afternoon from the Post Office. So we were all set.

The check came in from ATLFA the week of November fifth, and we called the dealer in Mechanicsville where we had the van on hold, to make arrangements to pick it up since we had the money.

We decided it would work on for Saturday morning, early, since it was my weekend off from work. Now we had to figure out who was going to drive either the van or our car back. Since Barbara had the accident in 1999, she wasn't comfortable driving in a lot of traffic or in places she wasn't familiar with. So we needed to find a second driver.

We thought about her uncle, James, but with his health problems didn't want to risk it. He was suffering with a bad case of bronchitis or something with his chest, and had been sick since taking his yearly flu shot the first day of November. So we called her aunt, (his sister) Annie to see if she would do it. She usually spends a lot of time putting out 1,000's of Christmas lights, but it happened she wasn't busy that weekend, and she agreed she would go with us.

A day or two before we were supposed to go, we got a call from Annie's daughter that she wasn't going to be able to go because her little dog had a medical emergency and had undergone surgery on one of her feet and had to be constantly watched.

Now we were in a scramble as to who we could find at such short notice. God is certainly good to us.

A friend of Barbara's from when she used to work in telemarketing back in the 1980's was online one night when she was on playing a game and they began talking. Barbara explained what we had to do on Saturday and we were trying to find someone who could drive the car or the van back. She said she wouldn't mind helping and all we had to do was to come pick her up at her house in Charlottesville.

We picked her up, and we joked and laughed and talked all the way down there. It seemed to make the trip go faster, which was a good thing. It also kept me awake and focused since I hadn't had much sleep since working past midnight Friday night.

When we got down there, I got a little turned around finding the place, but we finally got there.

Mary decided to stay in the car and smoke a cigarette while Barbara and I went into the building to sign all of the papers Steve (the guy who owned the van) had for us to complete.

We were in there for about 45 minutes, some of which was spent talking about NASCAR and how much we all enjoyed the sport. Finally, we came out with the papers and were ready to head home.

I decided I wanted to be the one to drive the van home and Mary and Barbara could follow me in the car. I didn't mind riding by myself, and figured I could turn the radio on to keep me company, and crack and window for a little fresh air.

To this day I haven't figured out how I got so turned around and confused when we left the car lot and started home. We ended up driving around and around in complete circles for over two hours, stopping—driving—stopping and driving, until I was totally frustrated, more than a little aggravated and my temper was definitely on a short fuse.

We finally stopped at a small little station and found out we had been going in the right direction the last time, but just hadn't gone far enough. Finally! We were on the road and I knew exactly where I was then!

We drove on up Interstate 64 toward Charlottesville without incident, or so I thought. It's funny though how things never seem to work out the way we plan or envision them.

A Jeep had almost side-swiped Mary and Barbara in the car and if it hadn't been for Mary jerking the wheel to the left he would have. Even another vehicle that was behind them had been blaring down on his horn to get the drivers attention, but he was too concerned with the conversation he was having on his cell phone to evidently pay attention to where his vehicle was on the road.

We stopped for a break and a bite to eat when we got to Hadensville Market. Sitting there, we enjoyed the food and soda and a break before leaving. When we pulled out, it was toward Charlottesville to drop Mary off before heading home.

Barbara would be ok driving from there to our house and all she needed was to have a few minutes to stretch her legs from sitting in the car for so long. She would also have to adjust the seat to suit her since she has short legs and the tilt wheel on the car doesn't move that far up to be very comfortable.

There was an event that was being the held the next afternoon that we had invited Mary to attend with us and we would pick her up after she attended church services.

Celebration of Life!

Barbara and I were both excited about the upcoming event: the Celebration of Life! at the University of Virginia; it would be my second one, and I was excited because I wanted Barbara to experience the camaraderie of the people who gathered together to celebrate the fact they had beaten cancer. It was scheduled the weekend of Veteran's Day, on November 11, 2007.

So many people had reserved a space they had to change the location from the hospital out to Alumni Hall on Emmett Street so there would be room for everyone.

We were a little late (doesn't seem like we get anywhere on time very often) picking Mary up at her house, and we went straight out to the University area. I wasn't exactly sure where Alumni Hall was located, but Mary had been asking around since her husband is working construction in the area, and she had picked him up from work.

We finally found it, only to be directed where to park by people with signs to attract those looking for the Celebration. I pulled over to the side at first, and walked to see where Barbara and Mary could find a place to sit so her wheelchair wasn't in the way, or she wasn't too crowded by people around her.

When I came outside, I unloaded the chair and Mary pushed Barbara inside while I went to park the van, and I would walk back from the parking lot.

By the time Mary and Barbara had stopped at the front table to get name tags and got inside, the worship service, being led by Chaplain Gordon Putnam was nearing its conclusion. They did get to hear a couple of selections of music and the closing prayer before it ended.

The banquet, prepared by University of Virginia Catering Services was a Thanksgiving Feast! Since it was close to the holidays, they had turkey with all of the trimmings, and luscious desserts galore!

The rest of the program consisted of updates for the new cancer center to shortly be under construction: UVa Emily Couric Clinical Cancer Center, scheduled to open in 2010, and named in honor of Virginia's late Senator Emily Couric, who was a former UVa Cancer Center patient.

The entertainment for the program was provided by Scott Burton, a well know comedian and juggler, who is also a cancer survivor. He has a wonderful comedy routine that mixes his experiences with cancer into it with a funny twist, providing much laughter.

We had the chance to meet and talk with him after the program, and he took several pictures with us before autographing a copy of his DVD and donating it to our support group, which was very generous.

We had the chance to talk to Gordon and Diane Cole outside the setting of the cancer center, and to meet her daughter, who also has red hair just like her mother, and a vivacious outgoing attitude. She was definitely having a good time!

Gordon and everyone who worked so hard to put the Celebration together did an awesome job. There were close to 400 patients, survivors and caregivers in attendance, and it seems to grow each year. We saw several of our support group members there, although Vikki had other commitments and was unable to attend.

Power Up!

We had the van parked out front and were now just waiting for the Scooter Store to deliver Barbara's power chair. It had to be special-ordered because Dr. Harper wanted a few special modifications made to the model she was getting, because of the degenerative bone disease.

He ordered legs rests, in case she needed her legs elevated instead of down on the footrest. He had also ordered an orthopedic back and special designed seat cushion that would prevent pressure points.

It would be delivered to our house from their office in Richmond, Virginia. Finally they called and said they would be there before noon on the following day.

Barbara did inform them we didn't have a ramp for them to use to get it in the house and they assured her it was alright since they brought portable ramps with them for that purpose.

Wouldn't you know it? The weather decided not to be very cooperative the following day. It was raining like it was coming out of buckets, but thankfully there was a reprieve when he unloaded the chair and brought it into the house. He did, however muddy the wheels because he had to go above the path we have from the parking area that has gravel. in

After bringing it into the house, we sat in the kitchen and he went over all of the warranties, parts and showed us both exactly what each part of the chair did and how to fold down the back, where the batteries (it has two) were located, went over the do's and don'ts for charging the chair, the guarantee, how to adjust the footrests, add the elevated leg rests, and any other important information.

With Barbara's short legs, he had to go to the truck and get the tools to adjust the rest so that it was more comfortable for her. Using a tape measure, he had to measure the main door ways in the house (kitchen, living room and master bedroom), for the paper work he would turn in to Medicare for payment.

Speaking of payment, Barbara's co-pay amount for the chair (the part not covered by Medicare) was a little over $900. Because of her limited finances (when she honestly told them that a payment plan would be a struggle), the Scooter Store had waived it, which mean that they took the loss, which I know they can write off of their taxes. I just thought that it was very generous of them to do that so that she could have the power chair.

He had Barbara sit in the chair and turn in around in circles to be sure she could safely and adequately operate it with the joystick. Then she moved into the living room to the opposite side, turned around and went back into the kitchen. The delivery man seemed satisfied with her ability.

Once he completed what seemed like a mountain of paperwork that she had to sign, he left her the copies she would keep and said if we needed assistance, not to hesitate to call the 1-800 number listed on the paperwork.

I Need a Lift!

Independent Lifestyles in Madison Heights had to order the lift they would be installing into the van and it would take about a week for them to get it from the manufacturer. ATLFA had sent them a copy of the check they had mailed me, so they knew we had received it.

Barbara talked with Josh and made arrangements to bring the van down there and leave it to have the lift installed, since it was at least an eight hour job.

Barbara's uncle James came over after he took his wife to work at Burger King he drove the Kia while I drove the van and Barbara rode with me. We didn't know exactly where we were going—just that it was right on Route 29 in Madison Heights. Barbara was a little familiar with the area since she and her first husband had delivered papers there when they did the route for his father-in-law whenever he needed a break from his route.

We were already on our way, and about five miles from home when it dawned on me that the check was still on our refrigerator under a magnet. Damn!

Since I needed gas in the van, and was going to stop at Sheetz a couple of miles up the road, I pulled off for James to do the same behind me. I got out and went back, handing him the key to the house and asking if he minded going back to get it for me.

We made pretty good time driving up there considering it was a long trip from where we lived. We stopped just outside of Amherst at a store that also sold hot sandwiches, to get something to eat and drink and to use the bathroom. James sat in the car while Barbara and I went inside.

Barbara asked him what he wanted and we brought it back to him. We sat there and ate before we left, and we laughed at this one vehicle—with junk piled high above the cab, and the guy who was driving looked like a mountain man that hadn't discovered what a razor or barber shop were. It was a combination of the Beverly Hillbillies and Sanford & Son!

Barbara was shocked about how much the area had changed since the last time she had been there, which had been a few years.

They now had a by-pass around the town, and we had to turn onto it to stay on Route 29, to go into Madison Heights, which also had grown. They had Home Depot, Wal-Mart SuperCenter, and several other national stores and companies now that used not to be there. We knew from Josh's directions that Independent Lifestyles was located just past Jiffy Lube, so that's what we kept an eye out for—finally seeing it in the distance.

When we got there, Josh went over the work order with us, and since everything else was in order, I signed the check (since they had made it out to me) and handed it over to Josh. Then we went outside and he looked the van over and described the work they would do to install the lift.

I had removed the bench back seat and stored it in my shed, in case we ever needed it. He assured us they would lock the van and that it would be locked into the back lot at night and on the weekends. We had loaded the power chair, since they wanted it to measure that the lift had been installed correctly, and he said they would charge it when they charged the ones they had on the premises belonging to them.

James had left his van (which is exactly like ours except its blue and ours is green) sitting in our driveway. When he got back, he gathered his oxygen and left heading home.

A couple of days before Thanksgiving we were supposed to go back and pick up the van. They had called and needed an extra day because the parts had been late coming in which threw them behind schedule by a day.

James went with us again, and got to relax in the back seat on the way down there. We stopped at Crossroads Market in North Garden for breakfast. Barbara decided to stay in the car while James and I went in to get the food. Well, at least I thought that she was going to stay in the car.

While we were standing in line waiting on our order she came inside to use the bathroom. I guess the cup of coffee she had before leaving the house was the cause of that. I left the line and walked her to the bathroom in the back of the store, and by the time we got back to the front, James already had the order and we walked out of the store.

When we got to the car, neither one of us had keys, and the car was LOCKED!! Now what the hell were we going to do?

When she had said she was going to stay in the car, I had tossed the keys down onto the console after taking them out of the ignition, and then went into the store. When she got out go in to use the bathroom, thinking I had hooked them onto the key strap I wear on my belt, she had locked the car without thinking. Her purse (and spare keys) was in the front floorboard. Now, here we stood with food in a bag and each of us with our tempers in an uproar, arguing in the middle of a busy parking lot! I went into the store and they gave me a flimsy coat hanger I was praying would work.

At least there was a small crack in the top of Barbara's window and this was one time that I was glad that she didn't like riding in an airtight car with the heat on. Maybe the coat hanger would slide down to the lock through that opening.

James and I both tried with no luck and I was getting madder by the minute, thinking we were going to have to call a locksmith we couldn't afford or Price Kia where we had bought the car for assistance.

James, somehow finally managed to pull the latch inside and unlock it that way. Because I had embarrassed her by yelling at her in public and in front of her uncle, she was a little ticked at me for the rest of the ride to Madison Heights.

When we got there Josh was busy working in the back so we had to wait for a few minutes for him to finish and to bring the van around to the front of the building.

Then he walked us outside and showed me how to work the lift. It looked simple enough. We spent another few minutes there, and then I got into the van with Barbara, and James waited for us to pull out so that he could follow us back home.

We drove straight through, not stopping until we were in Charlottesville and I had to stop at a gas station to use the restroom.

When we got home, Barbara asked me to carry James home since his wife had brought him over that morning so that she could use the van while he was gone with us. I took him home while she went into the house for something to eat and drink…

What a trip! Now, we had her mobility and a way to haul it. How we were going to get it in and out of the house and the van presented a whole new problem we would have to solve.

Constructing a Way

When we bought the van from Car Pro in Mechanicsville, it came with thirty day tags so we had a while before we would have to put tags, title and insurance on it.

Barbara had called our insurance agent and asked for a quote on how much our insurance premiums would be when adding the van, since we would need to put full-coverage on it because of the leinholder (ATLFA). We were both surprised to learn that it only increased the monthly premium thirty dollars!

I had some two-by-four boards which I used to move my lawn tractor in and out of the shed, and it was what I had used to take the power chair out of the house when we had taken it down to Independent Lifestyles. It had been awkward trying to move the chair on those boards, and Barbara and I knew that we needed to find a way to have a ramp installed.

We needed something permanent and stable to run the chair up and down on a regular basis.

Barbara's first call was to Construction Unlimited in Charlottesville. The owner of the business was also the Associate Pastor of our church, and she felt confident that he would give her a good deal on building a ramp for her since it was something that she was in need of.

She had been surprised earlier to learn that Sandy was now working for Steve in the business as Office Manager, and was not working for the Albemarle County Schools this year as a bus driver.

She talked with Sandy and explained what she needed and why, and Sandy said that she would give Steve the message and that he would call her back since he was out of the office at that time.

To this day she has yet to get the telephone call from him. Not only that, she called on several other occasions and still didn't get a response. She was disappointed, not just about the ramp.

We'd just have to look other places for that. What upset her most was the fact that things with the church had changed so drastically since Tommy had passed away.

In times past, whenever anyone connected with the church had said that they were going to do something it was like having money in the bank—you could count on it. Now, it was like their words didn't mean anything. Barbara, like me wasn't looking for charity or a hand out from anyone.

It was just that the church family we had means a lot to us, and to have them not even return a telephone call about something like a ramp—what, she wondered, would it be like if someone was seriously ill or on the verge of passing away? Would they not return the call for help? Not come to visit? It was very disheartening to say the least.

Barbara spent time on the telephone for over a week, off and on trying to find a way to get the ramp—and it seemed as if every place she called, she got the same answer—they didn't offer that kind of help, try somewhere else.

Finally, she contacted Rapidan Better Housing Authority in Madison, Virginia. They sent her an application which she filled out and returned to them the following day. She was already familiar with their organization.

Several years before they had done a lot of home repair for her mother—installing a bathroom and putting handicapped accessories in it, railings on her front porch; wiring the basement for her washer and dryer; putting light fixtures on the outside; installing electrical outlets outside; and several smaller jobs.

It had been under a government loan program, and if that was what they had in mind for us with building the ramp, we were both wondering where the money would come from to make the payment.

We were stretched to the max with the car and van payment and couldn't handle another bill, no matter how small it might be.

Cindy Reid, the Director of the organization called and wanted to come out and inspect the site and see what services they could offer. Our application had already been received and approved.

She came out and we sat at the kitchen table as she talked and asked questions to see what other services they also might be able to offer that would benefit her as far as her health condition was concerned.

Cindy and I used one of my tape measures and measured both the back and the front entrances to see which would be more feasible to install the ramp, and determined it would be safer and more economical to do it off of the lower back side.

Cindy said she had funds enough that she could buy the material if we knew someone who would be willing to do the actual labor. That way, it would prevent us from having to apply for a low-cost loan which she knew, after going over our income and expenses that we couldn't comfortably afford.

Barbara thought about her friend, Bill, who had said he could do it, and then thought better of it since he worked and there were other circumstances she didn't know about either. We were wiling to try and find someone and told Cindy that we would keep in touch. She promised to call and keep us updated on things on her end.

After several weeks, Barbara called and left message after message on her machine and never received a call back.

She was really aggravated, and one day she picked up the telephone and called the District Representative for Congressman Eric Cantor, Lloyd Lenhart and explained to him what was going on. He said that was much more manageable than trying to locate a van or other type of vehicle that would transport the power chair and that he would look into it.

Several weeks later, she received a letter from Congressman Cantor that he had forwarded the information to the Department of Housing and Urban Development for their review.

Barbara had several people make the comment that they couldn't believe she had actually called the Congressman's office about it. Well, evidently, they didn't know my wife! What was her response to them? Why not? He works for me!

Tom Aylor, owner of a construction company had stopped by and looked at the project and said that he would try to get it started before Christmas, and this was a couple of weeks before Thanksgiving. He didn't seem to like it very much when he found out that I work weekends on my job and would be unavailable to help with the labor.

Shortly after we received the letter from Congressman Cantor, a big truck delivered all of the material that the people would need to construct the deck!

The crew arrived on Tuesday afternoon, late—around two O'clock. They separated the lumber according to how it would be used, and dug the holes to set the posts. They worked every day that week, sometimes coming early in the day, sometimes in the afternoon. They completed the deck that week, on Friday at three in the afternoon and packed up everything to pull out! The ramp was built!

Healing Hands

I have been very fortunate throughout my journey through cancer to have a wonderful team of doctors and other healthcare personnel working closely with me every step of the way.

Everyone, including: my Surgeon, my Radiologist/Oncologist, to my Primary Physician and those in between. There of course, have been times when I was frustrated and angry that I felt I needed medical attention for various symptoms or problems that cropped up that I didn't receive, without having to go to either to my social worker or an R.N. in my surgeon's office to step on my behalf.

Some clinics just don't seem to get it. A cancer patient, after struggling through all of the treatments and dealing with so many adverse side effects tends to make us moody and not in the habit of being "put off", or scheduling appointments months down the road for something we're dealing with at the moment.

Every new ache, pain or symptom that we notice causes our heart rates to increase, we become panicky and immediately want an answer to what is going on—what can be done. We carry the thought of a recurrence in the back of our minds with every breath we take. And every little nuance of something in our bodies that isn't "right" scares the living hell out of us.

I've dealt with so many "other" things that have cropped up—all a consequence of either the cancer itself or the treatment to beat it, that I automatically call whichever clinic handles that particular part of the body. And, when they have the attitude of, "oh, well we can work you in to see someone in 3 months", it just doesn't work for me. The ones with attitudes like that do not seem to understand the hell that cancer patients have already endured and that when we call for help it is something that is needed right then, not months down the road, when postponing a check up could have even more devastating consequences.

I've had increased spasms, chronic dry eye, still deal with severe dry mouth, have had bladder issues (where they thought it was cancer and am still waiting to have a CT Scan done on the lining of my bladder), and other minor problems. I've had to make use of the position of staff in the Cancer Center to obtain the proper medical care for each of them.

One of the services that I applaud with great enthusiasm, and highly recommend to any cancer patient (whether they are still receiving treatment or have finished and in the survivor mode) that is offered by the Cancer Center's Integrative Medicine Program is the Massage Therapy.

Oh, the feeling of relief from stiffness and pain as the therapist's hands knead and work on muscles that don't get enough attention…its wonderful. I never about it until it was brought in one of our support group meetings, and trust me; I've taken full advantage of it. The therapist, Dinah McPerson Ray doesn't just work me over with her hands and ship out the door until the next appointment.

She asks questions, probes to find out how her service can be more targeted toward my individual need. She offers suggestions on other areas of my medical care that should be pursued or taken advantage of.

I think that all cancer patients could benefit from the application of massage therapy and would strongly recommend for them to check with their clinic or physician to see if it is available in their area. I am not just speaking from personal experience here, although it has done wonders for me personally. Massage, when administered by a licensed therapist provides two major benefits to the patient: first, it improves blood flow throughout the body and it also blocks signals of pain from nerves, tissue or muscles to the brain. It also releases the body's natural pain killers known as endorphins. It certainly is something that I look forward to each month, and it has helped me tremendously since I began receiving the treatments.

I deal with chronic pain in my neck and shoulders as a result of the lateral neck dissection to remove the cancer. The rehabilitation program provided by Larry Haywood was a Godsend to me to regain the mobility and use of my arm that was paralyzed and so weak after recovery that I could barely lift it to my waistline.

Get it up over my head? Absolutely NOT! But now, as I go into my 4th year out, the pain is often so severe it is breathtaking and sometimes stops me in my tracks. I tried going to the Pain Management Clinic, but all they could recommend was Cymbalta, which for some would solve the problem, but it was not something that I could ingest into my body, already depleted and having severe dry mouth as a result of the radiation killing the salivary glands.

For me, it made me drowsy where I didn't want to be active, and one of the side effects of it was dry mouth. Dry Mouth? Uh huh, I don't need help to dry it out, thank you. The loss of complete salivary function from the radiation does that all by itself. It doesn't need a helping hand. So, after taking several dosages of the Cymbalta, it went by way of the flush—straight down the commode and I was once again at square one. What else was there to try? Barbara, as usual went on a search mission to see what else was available, and after speaking with Diane Cole, Manager of the Cancer Center, suggested that I make an appointment with their Integrative Medicine Clinic to see what they had to offer that would be helpful for some of the side effects. It was certainly worth a try.

The staff of the Palliative Care Clinic has been wonderful to work with. They understand what I am going through with the pain and that I need something and the medication they have prescribed has worked been a wonderful balm to ease the pain and stiffness to where it is there and noticeable, but doesn't prevent me from doing what I need to do every day.

I still am careful what I put my body through physically, because I wouldn't want to do anything that would cause further injury or complications, and it definitely helps to have the medication to help out on days when there are things I can't avoid doing, whether it be on my job or in completing chores around the house.

There are some people who often associate Palliative Care with end of life, and that is simply not true, not entirely. Yes, they offer palliative care to patients who are terminal and there is nothing else that can be done medically to improve their condition or to lengthen the amount of time they have before imminent death occurs. This is the stage of palliative care where they use medications such as stool softeners or Tylenol for pain, or give sponge baths and turn the patient often to prevent ulcers (bed sores) from forming. However, Palliative Care is also used to help control pain and other symptoms after treatment for major illnesses and treatment, like with cancer. It is the goal of the staff in this setting to make the patient comfortable and that doesn't have to mean at the end of one's life, but aids them in living as pain free as they can as they live life to the fullest that they are capable of doing.

A Special Invitation

Barbara and Mark had worked so well together on a number of projects, and had become good friends, and I certainly liked him and respected what he had gone through and survived as a cancer patient and the work he was doing to help make a difference. He had an easy going personality and we all seemed to get along so well.

As the holidays approached, Barbara wasn't sure if Mark had any plans and we talked it over, deciding to invite him to come down and spend Christmas with us here at home.

Mark appreciated the invitation and they discussed the idea of him driving down, if that wasn't something that he wished to do, we were willing to prepare the dinner and drive up to his place in Maryland. It would have been a good outing, and would have given us a chance to drive the van and to try out the power wheelchair, as well. They finally set the date of December 27 for him to drive down, which we all agreed to.

We cleaned the house in stages, working methodically so that it wouldn't be very much to do at the last minute before he got here. We wouldn't do any of the cooking for Christmas Day or the day after since we were planning to visit family during that time.

We had finished our Christmas shopping a week or so earlier and had already finished wrapping everyone's gifts. Barbara made a chocolate cake to take to my mother, and brownies for my niece April and nephew, Joey for Christmas Day.

We enjoyed being with the family although Christmas is also a sad time for us. We were both thinking of our daughter Faith, who would have been just a week old that first Christmas we were together in 1998. I think of her each and every day, but the holidays are the worse.

Barbara not only had Faith in mind, but her mother, as well. Christmas had always been her favorite time of the year; and no matter how bad she was feeling, she always decorated with her lights outside, and a small dinner for the family, and I know it had been hard for Barbara since she'd passed away.

On Christmas Eve we traveled to Howardsville to have dinner with Barbara's aunt and the family. That woman is absolutely amazing. In her mid sixties and with a few health problems of her own, she has her house and yard looking like winter wonderland every year, with 1000's of lights and figurines on display. It takes her from mid to late October until a day or so before Thanksgiving to get everything staked out and hooked up. People will drive by and actually stop in the middle of the road to look at it. And the outside isn't all she does.

Inside she has lights strung in the living room, kitchen, dining room and hall, a tall Santa who greets with song and dance, and angels that wave from the window, where you can also see a beautifully decorated tree. There are over 75 Santa's on display on a special table she brings out of storage each year. It always makes you feel like you've walked into a special place.

She prepares a wonderful dinner with lots of food and this year was no exception. She prepared turkey, ham, turkey salad, rolls, mashed potatoes and gravy, potato salad, macaroni salad, stuffing, deviled eggs and a few other dishes, and for once we brought some home with us for the next day.

Barbara had already planned her menu for the meal she was preparing for us to share with Mark. She was having turkey breast, gravy and mashed potatoes, stuffing, cranberry sauce, a smoked picnic shoulder fixed with brown sugar and pineapple, green beans seasoned with bacon, deviled eggs, peach cobbler, sweet potato casserole, apple cinnamon cake, sugar cookies, oatmeal raisin cookies, orange balls and thumb print cookies.

Mark had told her that he prefers room temperature water with his meals and coffee after and she had that out and ready as well.

We had decided at Thanksgiving that we really were not going to decorate for the holidays this year. We hadn't bought anything, including a tree and were planning to wait until next year. But after we invited Mark, we got more into the spirit of the season and decided to go for it anyway.

One of our good friends, Peggy (not the one from earlier) got us a nice floor tree about 6 ft, and she also bought us a few new decorations, and loaned us some to go around the bottom of the tree that had belonged to her grandmother, which was very nice and appreciated.

I was still working in the CORE Lab at this time and had to go to work, but I went down and picked Peggy and her daughter Kayla up and brought them to the house, and Barbara was planning on taking them home later in the afternoon.

I have absolutely no patience with decorating a tree, and get very exasperated putting large ones like that together. Barbara is really good at decorating a tree, but with her back, it is hard for her to bend to do it.

Peggy and Kayla did an excellent job with putting it together and fully decorating it and I got to see it before I left for work.

Mark came down mid morning on the 27th and we all had a great visit. It was really nice being able to spend time together and cancer is not the primary issue or reason. He was very relaxed and I think he enjoyed it.

He is planning a trip to Africa next July with his sisters and their husbands, and he was telling us about things he needed to do to get ready for it. He has to have up-to-date shots, and has been looking at books on the country and area where they are going to be staying for the most part.

One of the subjects that he and Barbara have talked about is how they both enjoy cooking and baking. So after our meal, Barbara got out some of the cookbooks she's put together, along with the one that belonged to her paternal grandmother. Mark looked through them and actually found a couple of recipes he wanted, and made copies of them.

We had bought him a nice notebook organizer that turned into a "briefcase" if you extended the handles inside the pockets on each side. It was just something that we wanted to do and Barbara thought that since he is always going to meetings it would be something that he could use and enjoy. He was really surprised, and I think he really liked it.

He had rented a car to drive down for the day and had to have it back to the car lot at a certain time. It was a 2 hour drive, give or take a few minutes either way, depending on traffic on the highway.

Knowing we would be overwhelmed with all of the leftovers, considering we'd already eaten some of the dishes twice before today, Barbara gave him two containers to fill with whatever he would like to take home. He left around 3 O'clock with the promise to call and let us know that he had gotten home safely. It was really a special visit for us. Not only did we have the cancer in common, our goals to help others facing it, and had become friends. For him to drive down that far from home to spend a day with us meant a lot to both Barbara and I; and we really enjoyed his company, and was glad to spend time together.

We're Going Back!

I was sleeping so soundly when the alarm went off at 4:30 a.m. Groaning, I shut it off, and struggled to get my eyes focused as I put my feet on the floor, stretching before standing up, and moving toward the living room. Barbara was asleep on the sofa, so I went in to wake her before getting in the shower.

As the water cascaded over me I couldn't help but think we both had to be crazy to even think of traveling to Washington today. There was a major snow warning that had been issued, and it looked like it was definitely going to happen. We had watched the eleven O'clock news the night before, but didn't want to cancel the trip. It had taken a lot of planning to put it together, and Barbara would have been disappointed if she couldn't go.

When we had gone the first time back in August of 2007, Lindsay Shore had been nice enough to contact Congressman Cantor's District Office in Glen Allen, Virginia to let them know that we were interested in going on a tour of the Capitol, so they could make the necessary arrangements.

Lynnea Barrett, one of his staff members there called to schedule it shortly after that, but we decided to postpone making a commitment until after we found out if Barbara was going to be able to get a power chair or scooter. It had been too hard on me managing her manual chair on the first trip, and I didn't want to have to do it again for a tour.

Once we had the power chair, the van and the ramp had been built, Barbara telephoned Lynnea to schedule the tour, and the first date she gave us didn't fit into Mark Gorman's work schedule so we scheduled it for the day after, since he wanted to go with us on the tour and we had also scheduled a meeting with Lindsay for afterward.

As I showered, Barbara started a pot of coffee brewing before coming into get freshened up and to start getting dressed. Since we had no idea what the temperature would be like in D.C., she decided to wear a warm sweater and pants, with her Sketchers, which were not only comfortable but also had extra traction in case the weather got ugly and she had to step outside the van.

After getting dressed, we made sure we had everything we were supposed to be taking with us: cell phone, camera, Barbara's portable nebulizer, hair brush and license, along with a manila envelope she was going to get Mark to pass along to his former secretary who had retired at the end of December. It contained a lot of vegetarian cooking magazines she was looking forward to. Then we sat down at the kitchen table long enough to enjoy one cup of coffee each, before we left— knowing we would be pushing it to get to Congressman Cantor's office by ten O'clock—the time decided on for the guided tour.

Traffic on Route 29 doesn't seem to slow down for any reason, even impending bad weather. There were a few snowflakes falling as we got close to Madison, and yet there were several cars that zipped past us as if were sitting still. Sometimes it made me wonder how they ever got to where ever it was that they were going, because they didn't seem to care about anyone else on the road, and certainly not themselves.

When we got into Madison, we decided to stop at McDonald's and grab a breakfast sandwich and a drink to eat on the way. We would have preferred to sit and eat, but with the clock ticking, we knew we really couldn't afford the extra time.

Even though the time and miles seemed to go slow, we were on Route 66 leading to Washington before we realized it and the drive went smoothly, considering we were driving the van. It tends to make it pull and sway at times with the power chair and lift in the back. There were warnings posted on flashing "information" boards about a delay from Exit 60-64—which didn't bode well for us making it on time.

We arrived at the Vienna metro later than we had planned to be there but we were fortunate enough to find a parking space in the garage without too much hassle by going all the way to the roof area; we located one fairly quickly and it only took a few minutes for me to unload the power chair.

We had to travel a distance through the parking lot to the elevators which would take us to street level to go to the station itself. The power chair has a speed of about 5 miles per hour, but we couldn't use it because of the bumps how uneven the areas of the parking garage were.

We made our way to the station, with a cold breeze blowing and the temperature definitely had a bite to it, and Barbara complained her hands were freezing as she maneuvered the joystick on the chair. The sidewalks here were in remarkably good shape and we moved quickly inside. Before boarding the train we needed to find a restroom and to buy our tickets.

We remembered from our earlier visit where the bathrooms were located, but we needed a staff member to unlock the doors leading to it. So, we went inside where the ticket machines were located to find someone to help us. We are fairly new at using the metro and were a bit unsure of how to use the machines, so I found one of the station employees to help us.

The tickets cost a little more this time than on our first visit which surprised me. I was a little low on cash, and was worried about not having the correct amount, since they are unable to provide change for large bills, but we had enough. After we had our tickets, we asked to use the restroom, and he unlocked the door for us.

We made our way through the gates of the station and took the elevator down to train level where we had to wait for a few minutes for the next one to arrive. I had been worried about the power chair entering the train, but it went smoothly inside with no problem, and Barbara was able to maneuver it to where she was backed against a wall out of people's way.

Since we were not familiar with how to gauge all of the stops the train made, I sat where I could read the signs of all of the stations we stopped at between Vienna and ours at Capitol south. As it approached our stop, Barbara turned the chair on in to be ready to get off.

Mark was waiting for our arrival, and after shaking hands with me and giving Barbara a hug by way of greeting, we made our way up to street level to exit the metro.

We didn't have much trouble at first as we traveled down the sidewalks. But some of the brick have become dislodged or are missing all together, and some area's they are "humped up" which presented a definite problem for the chair. Barbara nearly turned it over twice and if it had not been for Mark and me, she'd never have made it over them without flipping the chair.

We entered Cannon House Office Building by going through the handicapped entrance, where we had to go through the routine security check. They allowed Barbara to move her chair around the security check where a guard used the wand to check her for weapons or other risks, and she was cleared to wait for Mark and me to finish with ours. I kept setting off the alarm and was finally cleared by the wand myself.

We made our way to the third floor where Congressman Cantor's office is located, stopping by a bathroom before going into his office. We were a short distance from his office when Lindsay Shore came to us in the hallway, hugging Barbara and I enthusiastically, so glad we were there; and finally realizing that Mark was with us, shook his hand before telling us to come on inside the office.

We were greeted warmly by all of the staff, and I know that Barbara felt out of place having to stay in the chair, which took up a lot of space, forcing people to step and slide around her as they moved back and forth inside. We were waiting for the person who would be our guide for the tour to get last minute instructions from Lindsay.

While we were waiting, we all removed our coats to leave them in the office, and I had to leave my water bottle as well because liquids aren't allowed inside the Capitol. Mark put Barbara's cell phone and my knife inside his bag and it was left there as well. We were all given name tags that we were to wear for the day and we were all set.

Our guide for the tour was Anna Kubit who hails from the Detroit area of Michigan, and who is working as an intern in the Congressman's office. It turned out, this was the first time she had led a tour of the Capitol, which should prove to be interesting.

She was vivacious, enthusiastic and very friendly so that was a plus. She kept apologizing because she didn't know a lot of information, but kept telling us we could ask other people in the areas we were visiting.

THE TOUR

One of the first things we saw on our walk to the entrance of the Capitol was a wall of pictures that had been painted by people who lived in each district represented in the House. One of the main winners was the painting from Virginia of a woman wearing a scarf tossed around her neck. It was a beautiful piece of artwork and was very detailed. There were workers busy preparing to hang more pictures as we walked by. The wall itself was located on the corridor leading to the entrance to the Capitol.

When we arrived at the entrance there were guards stationed and we were once again checked by security before being able to proceed. I could tell Barbara was excited about being there and was anxious to move on. It was really ironic that she felt that way now.

I don't know how many times over the years, when we were discussing different things, that she would say how much she hated the subject of government when she was in school, and how she often complained about why it was so important when she'd never use it in life. And now, here she was in the middle of the building that governed how our Government operates.

We saw the doors that had originally been made for the entrance to the Capitol but that were never used because they were too big. They had intricate carvings over the entire surface of the door. The doors were made of bronze which has aged to black over the years since they were made.

The bust of George Washington on display is the oldest known to exist and is the one that most resembled what he looked like. The original bust had been done by a sculptor from Italy, and a sculptor had recently refurbished them. This one was the most recent that had been redone.

Mark, using Barbara's digital camera captured two pictures of the bust to add to our collection.

We saw a miniature scale of Capitol Hill in a glass display case that Mark was able to capture a picture of in one of the area's, and we passed many statues of different influential members of history as we walked through the tour. They were located throughout the building, although the tour moved so quickly that we were unable to stop and read the inscriptions on each one.

We were taken to Statutory Hall, where prominent members of each state were represented with magnificent life size statues of their representatives and important people who influenced history.

Virginia has three statues: General Robert E. Lee from the Civil War, Thomas Jefferson and George Washington. Robert E. Lee, who we got a picture of, was the only statue on display in Statutory Hall, as Jefferson and Washington are in another room.

The next area was very beautiful and an important part of the "Capitol". It was the area that houses beautiful large paintings of different periods of history, prominently displayed along the walls throughout the room; where the statues of Jefferson and Washington are on display.

There is a Star in the middle of the floor that is the exact center of the Capitol. It is also the spot where they had originally planned to bury George Washington, but it was later decided that he should be buried at his home, Mount Vernon, Virginia. This part of the Capitol is known as the "Crypt."

The columns in the room are the original columns from the White House that was burned by the British during the American Revolution. They are "old" and charred, and have an important significance in the history of the United States.

The Dome of the Capitol is breath-taking to see. There are paintings in the ceiling that are absolutely magnificent, showing many different religious and other scenes. The colors are both vibrant and muted and very detailed.

The three areas that really impressed me were still to come.

One was the original Supreme Court.

Anna had to go find someone who could unlock a "lift" that would take her down to the bottom level where the Court was located, because the only entrance to it was down three steps.

Barbara had to back the chair in and then turn sideways while on top, which meant she was facing the opening when it reached the bottom level. She is claustrophobic, and said that she had held her breath and kept her eyes tightly shut on the way down.

It was the lowest portion of the first Senate Chamber in 1800. The Supreme Court occupied this space from 1810 until 1860. Most of the furnishings on display are original pieces, including six of the desks used by the justices. They are made of beautiful mahogany.

The large wall clock was made by Simon Willard and sets on the West mantel. It was ordered by Justice Roger Tanney in 1837 to be set five minutes fast so court started on time.

There are busts of 5 of the Supreme Court Justices placed throughout the chamber. They include: In the robing room: Roger B. Tanney (1836-1864); in the court room left to right: John Marshall (1801-1835), John Rutledge (1795); John Jay (1789-1795) and Oliver Ellsworth (1796-1800).

The room was the scene of many important cases including: Dartmouth College vs. Woodward in 1819, argued by Daniel Webster. In Dred Scott vs. Stanford in 1857, The Tanney Court ruled that a slave represented property and had no rights as an American citizen. The decision inflamed antislave sentiment in the North and contributed to the coming Civil War.

When the Court moved upstairs to a space vacated by the Senate, the room was used for a law library, reference library, a committee room and as a storeroom. Restoration of the Chamber began in 1972 and opened to the public in May 1975.

We then made our way to the Rotunda, one of the favorite places on the tour of the Capitol, and I admit it was one of most awesome sights I had yet to see on the tour.

It was unbelievably beautiful and I don't think that there are words to accurately do justice in describing the beautiful and very intricate work that went into the scenes that were sculpted around the entire circular dome. The sculptures depicted the original thirteen colonies of America, and major battles and conflicts, including the American Revolution, both World Wars, and others. We took several pictures with different views of it.

The height of the Rotunda is so great that the Statue of Liberty can stand in the center of the room and actually fit inside! Awesome and unbelievable to think that the magnificent "lady" could actually stand in the middle of our government and be a part of it; it was a very interesting piece of information to learn.

One of the things that caused me to pause and reflect for a moment on some of the recent things that have happened, was that we got to see where President Ronald Regan and most recently the body of President Gerald Ford had been when they lain in state before their funerals, where all of the officials in government and the public were allowed to file by to pay their last respects. It was a very special moment for me.

Barbara and I had closely followed all of the television coverage of the different ceremonies that were provided for President Ford, and to be standing within just a few feet of where his casket had actually stood to be shown the respect due to him for serving as our former Commander-in-Chief was a privilege.

Anna, being an intern and not very familiar with the layout of the Capitol (and I could well understand that because I still didn't think I could ever learn it because of it's size) got a little turned around a few times, and we had to ride the elevator a little more frequently than I know Barbara wanted to.

The elevators themselves were small, not normal size ones that you would find in places such as hospitals. The power chair takes up a lot of space, and even though it can pivot to turn tight corners it was hard to do once inside the elevator, and it was hard for her backing out of them into tight spaces.

We also saw the chandelier that was purchased by Jacqueline Bouvier Kennedy when JFK was President. It was absolutely gorgeous with what I would estimate as over 2,000 lights, and it was protected by a wooden barrier, and hung from the ceiling above an open area of the floor.

Our last part of the tour before returning to Congressman Cantor's office was "the Gallery", which is actually inside the US House of Representatives, which had a session going on at the time.

We had to go back to the security guards for a pass to go to the third floor of the Capitol which is where the Gallery was located, high above the floor of the House. We had to go through a very tight security check before we were allowed to proceed to that area. We had to check in our camera, cell phones, change and Barbara's envelope of magazines she had yet to give to Mark.

Then she was allowed around the walk through checkpoint, where she was checked by a female guard using the wand system. She had her small nebulizer with her as a precaution, and had to unzip it so that it could be thoroughly checked before it was placed back on her chair.

We were met at the entrance to the Gallery by the Sergeant of Arms, who opened the door for us to enter. It was a small area, circular in shape with chairs against the back wall and a brass railing in the front.

The area had a small closed circuit television where we could watch the proceedings that were happening on the floor below.

The floor of the House is awesome to look down on. The furnishings are a rich glowing mahogany and the carpet is a pale sky blue with designs in the middle. It was very moving to be allowed to watch elected officials debating a bill while we sat high above them listening in.

At the end of the tour we made our back to the Cannon Building and Congressman Cantor's office for our scheduled meeting with Lindsay Shore, stopping briefly for a soda at one of the vending machines along the way.

We waited for about half an hour before we finally asked if she were aware that we had finished our tour, and she immediately called us into the room, and we all sat around the table. We chatted for a few minutes, before Barbara asked where the Congressman stood on H.R. 1078.

Lindsay said that she still had some research to look up before he actually read over all of the material, and at this point we were glad that Mark had accompanied us into the room.

He was able to give her much needed information about it's scoring (which hasn't been done as of yet), but also on how many other private insurance companies are moving ahead with incorporating programs based on what this bill will actually provide for cancer patients and survivors. He had also prepared the information and left it with her which she said would greatly help her.

We left her shortly after that, Barbara and me both receiving hugs and we made our way out of the building. I think that all of us were feeling that the trip had been very successful and worth the journey to our nation's Capitol even on a day when the dreary weather outside would make it a slow ride back home I know all of our family and friends thought that we were absolutely crazy when we didn't postpone the trip when the National Weather Service had issued the travel and winter weather advisory's the night before, and I am sure we would hear more of those types of comments the following day when they telephoned us to find out how the trip had gone for us.

It was sleeting very hard as we came out onto the sidewalk. Barbara had quite a difficult time traveling back to the elevator for the metro, scraping against some of the bushes on the side in order to avoid the parts of the sidewalk with the worse places, and was glad to get to the elevator. Mark had an umbrella and was trying to keep it over Barbara's head as we navigated down the sidewalk but it was completely useless, and they both ended up soaked from the sleet that melted as it hit their hair and clothing. I was wearing my felt western hat, which was probably not the smartest idea in the world, but it did offer some protection against the stinging bite of the sleet to the top of my head. I was just hoping that the dampness left behind would not damage it or cause it to shrink or fade.

The trip on the metro from Washington to Vienna didn't really seem to take that long and there were times when it was a little crowded because it was toward the end of the day. For the most part it was a quiet and uneventful ride. One of the passengers did kind of get on Barbara's nerves a little, when he came rushing up the center aisle carrying a clipboard and very rudely bumped right into her as she sat in her chair and never said a word of apology, just kept going. A black lady sitting across from us said some people are such morons, and made a funny face by rolling her eyes skyward.

When we arrived at the Vienna station there was a really brisk wind blowing which made it feel even colder than the temperature actually was. We didn't waste much time going into the station and making our way up to the main level to leave. Barbara and I both needed to find the restroom because we had no idea what the traffic would be like once we got out onto the highway and our bladders might not wait until we found a restroom.

The metro stations always keep the big steel door that leads into the restrooms locked, because it is also the part of the building where their offices and supplies are stored in rooms. We had to find one of the employees who had a key and could unlock it for us. He was nice and friendly, and as we made our way out afterward, told us to have a nice day and a safe trip home.

Since the wind was blowing pretty briskly, Barbara took time to stop her power chair right inside the entrance to the open part of the metro station to light a cigarette. The sidewalks here were covered with both ice and snow and were pretty slippery; there was one of the employees using a small tractor to clear the sidewalks. At first I told Barbara to just wait right there and I would walk to the garage and get the van and come back to pick her up.

But when I started walking away from her, the sidewalks were a little more slippery than I liked and I said that maybe she should just come on and go with me. That way, I could watch out for her and hold onto the chair for traction and stability myself. I'm no fool! We made our way as fast as was safe to the garage. Mark had been generous enough to lend us his card to pay for parking so we wouldn't spend money out of pocket.

When we got off of the elevator at the top of the garage, the parking deck was snow covered with patches of ice in places, and we had to be careful. There were a few times before we got to where the van was parked that the tires on the power chair were spinning trying to find traction.

As we rounded the wall and the van came into sight it dawned on me that I hadn't bothered to bring an ice scraper with me and had no way short of using my bare hands to clean all of the snow off of the doors, windshield and top of the van so we could get in it and see how to drive. That was real bright, I thought to myself, especially since I knew that they had been calling for snow.

Mark had put the 2 copies of the story that he had printed for Barbara in the back pocket of the power chair and I got them out and laid them on the backseat while she was getting out and climbing into the van. I didn't want them to get wet because it was snowing pretty hard again, and they weren't inside of a folder or anything.

The roads there were in pretty bad shape that time of the afternoon and as we left the metro station I was driving slowly. As we got out onto the main road it really started coming down, and I had to turn the wipers on full speed so I could see where I was driving. I couldn't believe how some people were driving, like there was nothing on the road at all as they zipped by me like I was standing still, and I was actually going a little faster than the speed limit posted at the time.

Neither Barbara nor I had had anything for lunch and I was getting very nauseated and sick on my stomach because I hadn't had anything since the breakfast from McDonald's early that morning, except for sharing the Pepsi that I had gotten from one of the vending machines down the hall from Congressman Cantor's office.

We wasted a little time driving back because I took a couple of exits trying to find a fast food place where we could at least grab a hamburger or something quick to hold us over until we got home. Finally, we found another McDonalds' and stopped for supper, sitting there to eat instead of trying to do it while I was driving.

We stayed on the highway and didn't stop anymore until we got to Madison, VA where we pulled into the Sheetz so I could get a beer and a paper, and Barbara had to go to the bathroom. I got her a couple packs of cigarettes, and as we were getting ready to walk out, we ran into her cousin's husband, Charles. So we stopped and chatted with him for a few minutes before we got back in the van and drove the rest of the way home, checking the mail on the way into the trailer park. It was around 7 O'clock in the evening, and we were glad to have the trip behind us, although we were excited because it had been such a success, and we really had enjoyed our tour of the Capitol.

KAPLAN UNIVERSITY!

Barbara has never used her "trial period" under her Social Security disability. She did work briefly back in early 2000 before her mother got sick and down in the bed and needed constant care. But according to the SSA, because she didn't work over 3 months, it never counted against her. It means as of this date, she still has the full 9 month period, and can make as much income as she wants during that time.

She had never thought about using it because of the problems she has with getting around with the degenerative bone disease in her back. Not all of the places she might qualify for employment have wheelchairs that she could use to get around. However, since getting the power chair from the Scooter Store, it freed her up to begin thinking about it once again.

She really wanted to try to find a job working with people in the cancer center, because it was something that she was passionate about and had become quite good working with. She wasn't sure if they had any openings so she placed a call to Diane Cole one afternoon.

Diane thought that it was a great idea and was very enthusiastic and encouraging when Barbara told her about the idea she had. She checked but at the moment they had no openings. She also spoke with Dr. Michael Webber, Director of the cancer center. He encouraged her to check out the volunteer program and gave her the number for the director of the program.

After speaking with her and learning that she had no volunteer openings within the cancer center, Barbara decided not to pursue it because if she was going to do anything outside the home she wanted it to be gainful employment, so she could help pay some of the bills we had.

She eventually checked out the Medical Centers job website only to discover the jobs that were worthwhile were all for Medical Transcriptionists, and she didn't meet their qualifications. For a while she did nothing, and one day while on the internet she typed in Medical Transcriptionist—schools and a whole list of them popped up onto her screen. After wading through a few, the one Kaplan University Online caught her attention and she clicked on it and filled out the request for information page. Disconnecting, she went into the kitchen to start cooking supper, and shortly after that, the telephone rang.

The caller was Xavier Napier, who was one of the Admissions Advisors for Kaplan University! Barbara was shocked that she got a response from them so quickly, after assuming that they would send the requested information through the mail. They talked for almost two hours, and he said that he would call her back the following day and they could discuss things in more detail.

By the end of the week, Barbara had unofficially enrolled in the MT degree program for Medical Transcription, which is a 2 year program! Within 3 weeks, after a lot of telephone calls, faxes being sent, emails and attending seminars and going through filing applications for student loans and government grants, she is now enrolled full time, and her classes began on January 30, 2008.

Her first two classes were Academic Strategies and Medical Law and Ethics. After she had received her books by UPS on a Saturday afternoon and taken a look at the Medical Law and Ethics, she began having serious second thoughts about the decision to return to college. It was all so new to her and she was afraid that she wouldn't be able to keep up with all of the workload that the classes would require, but I tried to assure her that she had the determination that she would need to succeed. Ten weeks later, after hours of sitting in front of the computer, writing, rewriting and doing countless searches for information and material needed, she came out of her first term with not only a 4.0 GPA, but had actually been named to the President's Honor Roll for the first term! I think that it was only then that she actually breathed a sigh of relief, like she had been holding her breath for the entire time she had been in class. With her confidence restored, she began looking forward to her second term and I knew that she had found her niche and that she would be just fine.

An Unexpected Honor

Barbara and I enjoyed working with NCCS in promoting H.R. 1078—The Comprehensive Cancer Care Improvement Act on Capitol Hill, and it was something that neither of us in our wildest imagination ever thought that we would be doing. Barbara is more of the people type person than I am, and I have never been comfortable talking to people because of the speech impediment, and I am very self-conscious about it, especially around strangers. NCCS and the wonderfully dedicated staff who work there have done an amazing job of obtaining support for this piece of important legislation, and in late March, it was sent to the Senate side of Congress as bill S.2790. In mid April we received an unexpected package from NCCS that left both of us speechless and excited.

It was during that time that Barbara was spending a lot of time in front of the computer in the process of wrapping up her first term at Kaplan University. I came home from work at UPS (United Parcel Service) one afternoon and checked the mail on my way into the park. The envelope was addressed to both of us so I took the opportunity to open it while still sitting in the car, and had to read it twice to make sure I hadn't imagined the contents. NCCS holds an annual event that is a combination of a fundraiser for their projects and as a thank you for all of the patrons who have worked to make cancer a national priority. It is a very prestigious event with many key political figures, as well as those from the entertainment industry and the world of science and research. Inside the envelope was an invitation for Barbara and me to attend the event that was being held in Washington, D.C. on May 7th. I was shocked but very excited as I rushed into the house to share the news with Barbara, and couldn't wait to see what her reaction would be.

She was in her office wrapping up some research for one of the final projects that was due in Medical Law and Ethics, and when I handed her the envelope, everything else was forgotten as she read the information a couple of times, with her mouth literally dropping open and her eyes quickly scanning it several times. The list of people expected to attend the event was a Who's Who of Washington, news media and the entertainment industry all combined. Ted Danson of movie fame and the television show Cheers, Senator Ted Kennedy and his son, Representative Lois Capps (one of the sponsors for the CCCIA bill), Bob Scheiffer, news anchor for CBS news, Sam Donaldson, news anchor for ABC news, and Dan Abrams of MSNBC to name a few. The literature requested that we RSVP to a toll-free number to accept the invitation and Barbara immediately did so. Before the end of the conversation, she asked how we had received the invitation, and was told that it had been requested by Ellen Stovall, President and CEO of NCCS.

While the invitation was unexpected and something that we were definitely looking forward to, it did present some hurdles that we would have to overcome during the next couple of weeks in order for the trip to be a successful one. Our budget was tight and left little room for frivolities or unexpected purchases, like gasoline for extended trips or clothing, both of which was needed. The dress code for the event was business attire/cocktail and Barbara did not have anything that she felt would be appropriate for the event, and did not want to be embarrassed. Thankfully, the suit that I had worn to the event held in New York City would suffice for me, providing I had not dropped too much weight lately so that it still fit like it should. Barbara spent time mulling over what type of outfit she should try to find, and after speaking with Mark Gorman, opted for a dress since she wasn't very comfortable with pantsuits.

One of her best friends, Peggy said that she would start to look through some of her dress clothes and see if there was anything appropriate and that would fit her comfortably and we also began looking in different department stores in Charlottesville, which was easy considering most of them were holding sales for Mother's Day that was the following Sunday.

We spent over two hours in one of the department stores looking at all of the "formal" outfits, but with no luck. They were either not the appropriate size and there was not a wide variety to choose from. Peggy had several outfits but none that suited either, and we were fast running out of time to find something, when we found one at a Goodwill Thrift Store in Culpeper when we went down to grocery shop at the Wal-Mart SuperCenter. It was a black two-piece skirt set with white designs and black sequins on both the skirt and the top, and it was comfortable. Peggy had loaned her a pair of white heels and also a pair of black flat dress shoes and either would work with the outfit. Barbara retains a lot of fluid at times because of Peripheral Artery Disease, so it would depend on how swollen her feet and ankles were that day on which pair would fit comfortably.

The day before we were to attend the event, we drove down to Peggy's house late that afternoon and she cut Barbara's hair which had a lot of split ends and her bangs had grown down so that they hung in her eyes. After finishing hers, she also cut mine to give it a more uniform shape (mine tends to have "wings" at the sides that will stick out even when groomed). There was still a minor problem that we needed to find a solution to before the next day, since it would be late at night when we returned. We needed to find a "puppy sitter" for our 14 week old puppy Cheyenne.

When we moved into the trailer park, the landlord had been specific that he didn't allow pets (except for fish or hamsters that were in containers), and since we were only renting the lot and not one of his mobile homes, we couldn't understand how he could say that, but until recently we had abided by his "rule", even though we considered it stupid and unfair. All of that changed when we met Cheyenne. A friend of ours had a Dotson/Terrier mix that had given birth to a litter of pups and she needed to find homes for them once they were weaned from their mother. Sassy, the mother, was very friendly and would climb all over us whenever we visited, kissing and excited, and would bark, play and constantly climb into our laps for attention. She was also looking for a home once the pups were weaned and at first, we considered taking her since she was already grown and obviously attached to us. However, she had a tendency to bark quite a bit and so we finally realized that it wouldn't be smart, considering the rules of the trailer park.

Most of the pups were out and about which made it very difficult to walk in the house for fear of stepping on one. They were rambunctious and playful, allowing you to pick them up once in a while, but mostly they would roll around and loved attacking shoe laces and chewing on them. The "runt" of the litter stayed in the cage on the floor, very seldom coming out unless it was to use the bathroom, and was very shy and timid, and cold natured. She stayed toward the back of the cage where the baseboard heater was so she stayed warm. One night when we were down there, Barbara finally had the opportunity to hold her and make over her, and that was it! The puppy, shivering and shaking from probably being cold and scared, snuggled into her arms and buried her little nose in Barbara's neck and that was all it took. When we left our friends house to go home later that night, we had her snuggled into a thick towel and Barbara wrapped her coat around her to keep her warm.

It had been quite an adventure since then with the puppy. We discussed names all the way home, and still hadn't decided what to name her as we settled down in bed that night. Since we hadn't planned on bringing her home, we had no sleeping arrangements set up for her, and so Barbara laid her on her chest on the sofa and snuggled her under the cover the first night and that is where she still sleeps, unless she is in bed snuggled against me or under the cover in the middle of the bed. We finally settled on Cheyanne but every one spells it "Cheyenne". She is totally spoiled now, and most people laugh because she has toys, treats and a baby blanket that is her "security" and she won't leave home without it. Peggy finally said that she would keep her overnight for us and that we could come and pick her up the next afternoon.

I took off from work that day so that we would have enough time to prepare for the trip without feeling rushed and tired by the time the event started later that evening. We gathered all of Cheyenne's things together that she would need for the overnight stay, showered and dressed, and gathered things we would need. Peggy had found two nice skirt sets at a local yard sale for Barbara and she wore one for the trip to D.C., and took her outfit for the evening in a bag. She had decided to wear a formal evening dress that she had purchased from Sears a few years before when we had been in the Herbal Life Organization. It was a multi-colored sequined gown that was "dressy" but would pass for a cocktail dress. We arrived at Peggy's a little after two in the afternoon, and she styled Barbara's hair and did her make-up for the evening so that all we had to do was stop before arriving so that she could change into her gown, and touch up her lipstick. I went to McDonald's and bought the chicken wraps for lunch and we ate at Peggy's before saying goodbye to Cheyenne and driving off, with her whimpering of course.

We talked on the drive up to Washington, and were pleasantly surprised that traffic was light and not difficult to navigate, even as we got closer to the city. However, on the other side of the interstate, it was a different story. There was bumper-to-bumper traffic coming out of the city, as people left the central nerve of our government behind for the more relaxed atmosphere of the suburbs of Northern Virginia. I was very thankful that it would be much later in the evening before we would be leaving and hopefully, by then it would once again be light traffic to maneuver on our drive back to Orange Virginia.

When we arrived in D.C. we found Constitution Avenue without any problem, except I drove right past the building and had to turn onto Pennsylvania Avenue to turn around and go back. What a nightmare! The traffic was bumper to bumper, and there was no courtesy to each other at all. We waited for over fifteen minutes for a break that would allow us to make the turn without any success. I finally drove down another two blocks to turn around and head in the right direction. We parked on the side of the street so I could find out about the valet parking that was supposed to be available for the event. One of the dressed valets assured me that at 6:30 we would be fine exactly where I parked because we had the handicapped car tags, and had put her manual wheelchair in the trunk of the car.

After helping Barbara get settled into the wheelchair, I secured the car and turned on the burglar alarm before we started down the sidewalk in search of someone who could help us locate the handicapped entrance. There were several people standing around in "uniform" dress and as we approached, a young lady disengaged herself and came toward us. She led us toward the back of the building and down the alleyway where the catering service was set up to prepare the sit-down dinner later in the evening, and it took approximately twenty minutes to locate the entrance and gain access, which was totally frustrating for both Barbara and I. They were evidently not equipped to handle a guest who was in a wheelchair, and Barbara had to get out of the chair, walk several small steps and then sit back down in order to get inside. By that time, half of the cocktail reception was over.

The room was very crowded and it was more than a little awkward for us since we didn't know anyone, and Barbara immediately suggested that I leave her where she was sitting in a small space and go in search of Mark Gorman or Dan Waeger who were the only two members of the NCCS staff that we had met at that point. I went to the bar set up at the end of the room and got us two drinks and then left in search of them, which was hard to do with wall-to-wall people milling around in conversation.

Barbara's View:

I was totally frustrated by the ineptness of the people who were responsible for working the event in helping us get inside the building just because I was using my wheelchair. I like to be punctual to anything I am supposed to attend, and since we were invited by the national group, I just felt like we owed it to them to be on time, and we had worked so hard on our end to allow time so we wouldn't be late, only to have these people make us late.

I was anxious anyway, having never been around so many political people in my life, and didn't like the fact that we had not made arrangements for someone we knew to meet us at the entrance, and now we were totally on our own. As we entered the room where the cocktail reception was being held, it was hard to move more than a foot or two at a time because it was so crowded. As my eyes rapidly scanned over those standing around, I knew that locating Mark or Dan would be like looking for a needle in a haystack, and it was quite obvious that Dwayne would not be able to maneuver my wheelchair around in the crowd. I assured him that I would be fine where I was until he tried to find them, and watched as he began making his way through the people and move away from me.

I had the opportunity while sitting there to meet several members of the board of directors for NCCS and their spouses, and enjoyed conversing with them. Sam Donaldson entered the room and I was able to speak with him for several minutes. He is one of the outstanding reporters for ABC News and he himself is a survivor of melanoma. I was a little bit at a loss for words when Senator Ted Kennedy came into the room and introduced himself to me, and shaking my hand.

Like most Americans, I had followed the lives of the Kennedy family for years, through all of their political triumphs and family tragedies, including the death of John Kennedy, Jr. several years earlier in a plane crash. Senator Kennedy is a member of the Senate Health Committee and a staunch supporter of not only NCCS (with whom he has worked closely) but cancer research in general, and the passage of key legislation for cancer care in the United States.

Dwayne returned about twenty minutes later, having had no luck in locating either Mark or Dan, and we decided to make our way to the back room where NCCS had their board established for picture taking. It was a little tricky trying to maneuver the wheelchair through the crowd and we spoke to everyone we asked to move, making our way there after about ten minutes. The room was pretty vacant, with different ones wandering in and then leaving again, and we were preparing to leave as well, when I spotted of all people, Lance Armstrong!

When I pointed him out to Dwayne, his reaction was: "Are you sure it is Lance Armstrong?" I did a double take, looking at him. How could I not know Lance Armstrong? I had seen him countless times when the Lance Armstrong political forum had been televised, on lots of commercials, his website, and the hundreds of pieces of literature categorized on my wall shelf at home. Of course I was sure it was Lance Armstrong! Dwayne eventually followed him out of the room to ask if it would be possible to have our picture taken with him, and when he came back he told me that Lance had said to come back in a few minutes after a speech he was interested in had concluded. I wasn't about to pass up that opportunity, and so we began making our way to where he was engrossed in a conversation with several gentlemen while trying to listen to a speech being made at the front of the room.

Dwayne's View:

I was really surprised at how small in stature Lance was in person. It appeared that while his body was well-honed and maintained, he was short in comparison to most of the athletes I knew, and his weight was probably something he worked to maintain as well. He was open and friendly, and it felt as if we were talking to a friend or neighbor whom we had known for years. He was glad that we were there to help NCCS celebrate their success and thanked us for supporting cancer and research. I was able to tell him a little about the type of cancer that I had been through, and he clasped my hand in a warm, friendly handshake to congratulate me on joining the ranks of survivors, he being one of testicular cancer. Barbara and I both took the opportunity to express our gratitude to him for his foundation awarding us the full travel scholarship that will allow us to join in participating at the Summit to be held at Ohio State University at the end of July, and we let him know how much we were both looking forward to being there.

As the conversation ended, so too did the cocktail reception as people began making their way toward the dining area for the sit-down dinner. We were assigned to tables so we asked workers who were seated at a table in the back room to help us locate the table where we would be sitting. The tables were arranged throughout the room, and unfortunately it would have been very awkward to try to get around them with the wheelchair. A gentleman offered to help us locate the table and was willing to rearrange the chairs for me to push the wheelchair through them, but Barbara, being resourceful, opted to walk to the table and so we folded up the chair and found a spot to place it so that it wouldn't be in the way of foot traffic. As we made our way to table #25, we couldn't help but notice how beautifully decorated they were.

Each table had been arranged for nine guests to be seated, and each had beautiful flower arrangements in ceramic vases of different shapes and colors. The table was covered with a peach or green tablecloth, matching napkins, a large plate that dinner plates (for each course) would be placed on, wine goblets and water glasses made of crystal. After we had taken our seats at the table and were looking around the room, Mark walked up behind Barbara, speaking to her over her left shoulder, which caused her to jump in surprise. It was nice to discover that he would be seated at our table, so we knew at least one person. He took the time to introduce us to the people seated to our left and our right, both of whom were members of the board of directors for NCCS. I think that both of us were nervous because we had never been to such a formal dinner before and it felt a little awkward at first. I am somewhat self-conscious about eating in public since the surgery, and it takes me a while to eat because of the problems with my dentures.

The first course was a spring crab salad, and was a dish that neither of us had ever had before, and I knew that Barbara wouldn't enjoy it because she doesn't like seafood that much, and will only once in a while eat shrimp. I didn't know what it was, thinking that it was some sort of tuna dish until Barbara whispered what it was. Actually, once I began eating it, I found that it was very good, although I noticed that Barbara only made a gesture of enjoying hers, washing it down with the wine that the waiters kept the glasses filled with. After she noticed that Mark didn't finish his either, she delicately laid her silverware down, pushing it aside, and turning to speak with her dinner companion.

The second course was much more appetizing and appealing. It was beef tenderloin in wine sauce, with fingerling potatoes and spring green beans with butter sauce. It was very tender and juicy, with just the right amount of spices making it favorable but not overpowering. The only frustrating moment came when I didn't have the chance to finish all of it before the waitress arrived with the baked Alaska for dessert and I had to let them take it. Damn! I wanted it but if I had kept it I would have missed out on dessert, and I certainly didn't want to embarrass anyone, including myself by making a scene. As the wait staff wrapped up serving the dessert, Dan Abrams, anchor at MSNBC began addressing the crowd during the opening part of the awards ceremony, introducing Ellen Stovall, President and CEO of NCCS, who welcomed everyone with a short speech. She talked about the early years and how NCCS was founded in Albuquerque, New Mexico, her diagnosis of cancer 37 years prior, and the work that she has managed to accomplish with the organization, and also about her recently discovered recurrence, and the fact that she will be stepping down at the end of 2008, turning the reigns over to her successor, who still has to be found. She also took the time to acknowledge the members of the board, as well as having members of NCCS staff stand for recognition as well. It was nice to see that Mark has worked his way into position on the staff since he first began as a volunteer with NCCS after his treatment for cancer and has definitely come a long way.

There were multiple awards given, with the most prominent ones being: Bob Scheiffer of CBS News for media coverage, Sam Donaldson for his work with promoting cancer, and the most special was the presentation of lifetime achievement award to Ellen Stovall for her work and dedication on behalf of cancer patients, survivors and caregivers for the past 20 years. It was very touching when to make her acceptance speech, her family joined her on stage.

Barbara had been sure to take her trusty little digital camera, with new batteries along to take pictures of the event so that she would be able to share them with the members of our support group at the next meeting. However, Mark came over and told her that they would be getting copies of everything from the professional photographers that they had on hand for the event, so that the only picture we took was the one with Lance Armstrong, and one of the Washington Monument on our drive into town. He asked us to stay around at the end of the event so that he would have the chance to introduce us to the rest of the people from NCCS and we were definitely looking forward to that.

Barbara had been instrumental in getting to know most of them and would share all of the news from the telephone calls with me when I came home. She was shocked when she finally met them because they were nothing like the mental picture she had conceived of them, and was pleasantly surprised by how friendly and down to earth each and every one of them were. It was definitely an honor and a privilege for both of us to be among other survivors who had taken their experiences and turned it into a way to spread help to others facing this devastating and life changing illness, but to show that life indeed can go full steam ahead after treatment, and that the experiences we go through can be turned into positive and worthwhile work, and not be something that we are ashamed of or that we should sweep under the carpet like it never existed.

SUMMER CAMP 2008

When Rapidan Better Housing Authority had come into build the original wheelchair ramp for Barbara's new power chair, they only build the ramp itself, and the two side rails the length of it, since their funding was in short supply and didn't allow for extra's. However, when the work was complete and Cindy Reid, the Director of the program came out to do the final inspection, she mentioned a group of people who were college students and other young volunteers who might come out to do some other work that was needed to our mobile home in order to make it handicapped accessible.

Several weeks later, members of that group came out to inspect the house and find out what we felt we needed in order for Barbara to be able to maneuver the chair throughout the house without having problems. They looked at each area, took pictures and made notes and said that they would be doing the work sometime toward the middle part of June after school was out for the summer vacation.

It turned out that the group was from Arlington, in Northern Virginia and was part of the Archdiocese of the area, and were all volunteers—from college students to teachers, police captains and others, who used the program to not only help those less fortunate, but to learn a trade that would be useful in life, and to learn the true meaning of giving and sharing with others. The group that came to our house was made up of 9 young men and women and was accompanied by an adult leader skilled in the area of work that they would be doing. They were to extend the deck approximately ten feet to make loading the chair easier, add pickets to each side of the railings to improve the looks and value of the project, widen the master bathroom doorway so that the chair would access the room, raise the commode to make it easier for Barbara to use, modify the shower with a hand-held shower unit and a portable bath bench for safety.

Madison Wood Preservers delivered all of the lumber and hardware accessories needed on Friday mid morning, and they came ready to work on Monday morning. They all came in to introduce themselves and let us know the hours they would be there, and they provided their own lunch and snacks for break time, although we had made the arrangement prior to the start date that we would prefer that they use our guest bathroom instead of having the portable toilets delivered and set up on the lot. Our landlord is a very strict person who can be very difficult to deal with at times, and we in no way wanted to make any waves with him while having the work done.

All of this was taking place at a very difficult time for us financially. We had our car repossessed by Wachovia Dealership because I was between jobs and we had gotten behind on the payments, and since the Stimulus package that we were supposed to be getting from the Federal Government would not arrive in time to help out; there had been little choice except to let them take it back. This meant that the only transportation we now had was the Grand Caravan which used a lot more gas and cost more money to maintain than the car had. When Allied Janitorial began cutting my hours back from 25 to 15, and with the steady rise in gas prices, I knew that I would have to begin looking for another job, and was scheduled to begin working at Klockner

Plentaplast Plant in Gordonsville that very week. However, it presented major problems with not having money to purchase gas and we were running very low on food supplies and staples.

Barbara was on the telephone a lot that week calling various organizations all over our community trying to get help not only for food and gasoline, but the bill for electricity that we had received a shut off notice for the following Monday. It was indeed a very stressful time for both of us, but God always provides a way for those who have the Faith to rely on Him for their needs. Not only was the light bill paid on time to prevent interruption of service, we received meats, fruits, vegetables, microwaveable dinners, and household supplies from various churches and organizations in the area, including a gas card and a tank of gas for the van from two separate churches. It was indeed a true Blessing and one which we praised and gave Him all the honor and glory for.

The group of young people was very dedicated and hard-working. They did a remarkable job on finishing all of the projects in a timely manner, always cleaning up each day before leaving, and it was with a bit of regret that we said goodbye to them late on Wednesday afternoon. We have a framed picture of the group, signed by each of the as a memento of the time we spent together, which we have proudly displayed in our living room. We were truly blessed to have been touched by their caring, loving attitudes and smiles during the time they were here with us, and it made the days quite enjoyable for both of us.

We wish them all the best in future endeavors.

Preparation for the Summit

Barbara was very vocal in advocating for quality cancer care with the people at National Coalition for Cancer Survivorship and was a subscriber to the Lance Armstrong Foundation's newsletter to keep informed about events and issues that might be of interest to patients at the Cancer Center and our support group. We were delighted that our efforts on Capitol Hill had paid off when the Comprehensive Cancer Care Improvement Act was submitted to the Senate earlier in 2008 and we are looking forward to visits with the Senators from Virginia to discuss its merits and advantages.

In February of 2008, an email from the Lance Armstrong Foundation alerted everyone to sign up for the 2008 Summit to be held in July on the campus of Ohio State University in Columbus. Barbara and I discussed it and thought that it would be an advantage in attending, so she filled out the necessary information, requesting scholarship because of our limited income. We were hopeful that we would be chosen to attend but didn't spend a lot of time thinking about it because we were both busy with work, chores around the house and Barbara was swamped with all of the research and writing assignments for Kaplan University.

When the email arrived informing us that we had been chosen as Virginia delegates to the Summit we were delighted, but when she shared the news with Mark Gorman at NCCS, he was skeptical about our attending, and thought that Barbara could afford to skip it and concentrate on her school work since the trip would come on the heels of her third term starting, and two of the most difficult classes to date with Anatomy & Physiology I and Software Applications, both requirements for her degree program. We did give it serious thought but decided that we would attend. LAF (abbreviated) was doing the same type of work as NCCS and we thought that combining the styles of the two premier advocacy organizations in the country would help when we were meeting with elected government officials on behalf of cancer patients, and give us a clear picture of the needs and how to approach them for help.

The dress code for the event was casual so we didn't have all of the hustle and frantic searching for the appropriate clothing that we had experienced when we were trying to prepare for the dinner in Washington with NCCS, although Barbara had bought some nice summer pants that would have been nice. Unfortunately, whenever she finds the right size they need to be altered to be the appropriate length and we didn't have the extra money for a tailor or enough time for anyone we know to get them done before we were to leave on the trip. We each chose outfits from what we already had available in our limited wardrobe and didn't worry about it.

We did have to find someone who would be willing to keep Cheyenne during the time that we would be gone since we wouldn't be able to leave her at home alone from the 24-27. We decided that since Frances Payne (whom we had gotten her from) had her brother Peanut and 3 cats that could keep her company, it would be the best place for her, and Frances agreed that she would keep her. It was the first time since we had brought her home that we would be away from her for any length of time and we knew that we wouldn't like it anymore than she would. She is totally spoiled and not everyone will let her get by with some of the things that Barbara and I do, and we knew that Frances would definitely have her hands full.

I had started a new housekeeping job with The New Company of Virginia located in Charlottesville and was working at Klockner Plentaplast, located in Gordonsville, Virginia—about a 15 minute drive from home. I was lucky to get the job there, and it definitely cut down on both the travel time to and from work as well as the cost of gas since the explosion of oil prices had driven a lot of people to seek public transportation or to start biking to work. After solving the clothing and dog sitting issue I had one more hurdle to get over before the trip. I had to convince my employer that I needed to have 2 days off, since we would be leaving early on Thursday morning and not due home until late in the evening on Sunday. I had been sure to mention the trip to him when I had first interviewed for the position, and at that time he had assured me that it would be alright, but now I needed to remind him beforehand. I should have known that someone would throw a monkey wrench into the preparations and that it wouldn't go as smoothly as I wanted it to.

I was due to receive my paycheck the Friday after we departed for Columbus and I wanted to work it out so that I could either pick it up late Wednesday afternoon, or at least by 7 am on Thursday morning before heading out to the airport. I was told that in order to ask for the check and for the two days to be approved, I had to file a request of leave form with the main office of the company. I brought the paper home and Barbara helped me fill out the information and I took it to the main office when I got off work the following day. I was told that they would let me know their decision by the following Tuesday, but they didn't see a problem with the request. Wrong. When I finally got in touch with my boss on Wednesday instead of Tuesday, he said that yes, I could have the time off from work for the trip but that he couldn't authorize my getting the paycheck until after I returned because of the way the time went into the payroll department! What a crock!! Now, what the hell were we supposed to do for spending money, since we would have to provide our first meal at the Summit on Thursday night and any incidental expenses that we would have while in Columbus? We had been playing catch up with all of our bills and had not had the chance to save any money either from Social Security or from any of my previous paychecks, and it was unfortunately looking more and more like we would have to turn down the trip after all. We could risk over drafting our bank account until the first of the month, but then it would shorten the amount we had for the bills due at that time. Finally, Barbara—in a last ditch effort to avoid cancelling out, called Vikki Bravo.

Barbara asked her if we wrote her a post dated check for the following Tuesday if she would be willing to lend us $100 cash for the trip and then she could deposit the check the day after I went back to work and could put the money in the bank to cover it and thankfully, she agreed. I came home from work on Wednesday and Barbara, leaving Cheyenne at home since it was so hot outside, went with me to Charlottesville, where I paged Vikki from the lobby of Hospital West. She brought the envelope out and we spoke to her for a couple of minutes, since she was still at work, and received a hug and wishes for a safe trip. We still had one more stop to make before returning home. Ellen Desper, another angel that we have had the pleasure of becoming friends and working closely with, had made arrangements for us to meet her at Rent-A-Center at the Rio Hill Shopping Center where she was going to pay for us to rent a laptop computer so that Barbara would not fall behind in the assignments for school while we were gone. When Barbara had asked her if she knew anyone who could loan her a laptop, she had had no idea that when she wasn't able to find someone, that she would actually rent it herself. It goes to show that you can always expect the unexpected in life.

We did not want to have to get up so early on Thursday morning and drive to Frances' house in Fork Union, Virginia which is about 50 miles one way to drop Cheyenne off before hustling back to get to the airport on time. We were scheduled to fly out at 11:15 a.m., and needed to be there for check-in at least an hour prior to that. When we left Rent-A-Center in Charlottesville, we stopped at Sheetz convenience store in Ruckersville to top off the gas tank and to purchase cigarettes for the trip before going back home. We sat down and had something cool to drink and packed up all of the things that Cheyenne would need for her stay, including her bed and blankets, toys, shampoo, bones and food, before leaving again for the drive to Frances' house.

We had told her on a previous visit that we would be coming over to drop Cheyenne off the night before we left so we naturally assumed that she would be home and everything would go off without a hitch—boy, did we get a surprise! By the time we had finished all of the other errands that had cropped up unexpectedly, it was getting late into the night by the time we got to Fork Union. The weather sure didn't cooperate and we had to stop several times during the drive because torrential downpours made it virtually impossible for me to safely drive due to very limited visibility. We pulled into her driveway it was just shy of 10 pm and there were no lights on in the house, although her car was parked in the driveway, so we knew she was at home. Thankfully, the rain had yet to start there, so I told Barbara to keep Cheyenne with her and stay in the van while I went and knocked on the door. She didn't have the outside light turned on and I didn't want to take a chance that Barbara might fall and hurt herself trying to walk to the front porch. I spent about ten minutes knocking on the door and nobody answered it. We were really in a pickle if we couldn't leave Cheyenne there because we didn't have anyone else to keep her. Finally admitting she wasn't coming to the door, we left and went to Peggy's house in Scottsville where Frances' son, D.J. had been spending time with Michael, Barbara's nephew since the 4th of July. We thought that perhaps Frances had taken sick and was back in the hospital or maybe she was there at Peggy's visiting with her dad.

What's the old saying, "if it weren't for bad luck, I'd have no luck at all?" Well that old clique certainly seemed to be following us around tonight as I pulled away from Frances' house for the drive to Peggy's. Almost as soon as we were back on the road, the heavens opened up and another torrential downpour began, which meant that I was driving at a snail's pace one more time. We had been lucky before because it seemed to come in spurts. This time, however it didn't seem like we would be lucky enough to catch a break, and when we finally pulled into Peggy's driveway, it was raining like cats and dogs.

We sat in the van for a few minutes waiting for it to let up before trying to get out and onto the front porch of the trailer. We didn't need to wonder if anyone was still up that time of the night because nearly every light in the house was on, including the front porch light. Finally, we made a dash for it, with me carrying Cheyenne since I was surer of my footing and could move faster than Barbara. I was trying to keep her from getting soaked to the skin and running the risk of her getting sick and needing to go to the veterinarian, since it was an expense that we couldn't afford right now. When I knocked on the door, Peggy answered and wanted to know what in the world we were doing out on a night like tonight.

We would much rather have been at home out of the nasty weather and getting ready for bed, since we had to be up and ready to go fairly early, and it would definitely be a long and exhausting day by the time it was over. I asked her if D. J. was there, and he came to the door. I explained that we had just come from his mother's and that we couldn't get anyone to answer the door and I thought that maybe she had gotten sick or had decided to come up to spend time with her dad for a while. He called the local hospital where she always went for treatment if she got sick and she had not been there. He asked if there were any lights on in the house. I told him that there hadn't been any, that her car was parked in the driveway, and that the air conditioner in the living room window was running. He had a key to the house with him and he offered to ride down there and go in to see if Frances and his sister Elizabeth were alright. I should have known that it would not be a simple thing when he suggested doing that—which was just the way our luck had been running for us all day long.

Michael, the oldest of Peggy's grandchildren wanted to ride along, and D.J. said that once he found out what was going on down at his mother's he wanted to come back up to Peggy's and stay, which meant it was going to be even longer before we were actually back home and could get some sleep. We never did go in the house which was really crowded. A lot of teenagers that were friends of Michaels and his brother and sister were inside, and it was noisy, with music blasting from different areas of the house. It was a good thing to stay outside on the front porch, where Barbara made herself comfortable on the swing. We wouldn't have been able to have a conversation or even hear ourselves think inside anyway.

We talked to Peggy for a while, and Bill finally ventured outside as well, to talk to us as we waited for D.J. to find clothes and socks to go with his shoes. I hadn't taken the time to eat any of the chicken that we had stopped at Hardees's in Gordonsville to buy on the way through, so I went out to the van to eat and finish my drink while waiting. Barbara was still sitting on the swing holding Cheyenne, because we were afraid that she would take off running into the rain, and since she is black and it was night, were concerned that if she got loose we would have a devil of a time finding her again. Finally, we were ready to leave.

Barbara asked D.J. if he would carry Cheyenne under the hooded shirt that he had slipped on to stay dry and he took her and made a dash for the van. I had planned on coming back to the porch with the lightweight jacket that we had in the van for Barbara, but she had her own ideas. She made a dash for the van, and was as wet as a rat by the time she got into the front seat. Both D.J. and Michael were more than a little peeved and complaining because I had told them that they couldn't smoke while riding in the van. Barbara smoked, but since there were no ashtrays in the van and we had to use the window, we couldn't let them. The windows in the back do not open and we couldn't have opened them anyway with it raining like it was.

I had to drive slow because the rain was really pelting down and whenever I met another vehicle on the road it was really hard to see. It took about twenty minutes or so before we finally pulled into Frances' driveway again. We waited inside the van while Michael and D.J. got out and went to the front door. After knocking and getting no response, he used his key to get inside and shut the door. We took the time to talk to each other while we were waiting. After about 10 minutes, we finally saw a light come on in both the living room and the kitchen, and D.J. finally stuck his head outside and told us to come on inside.

Everyone was in the kitchen when we walked in and we felt kind of strange being there that late at night. We took turns using the bathroom and found seats in a couple of the chairs, and Peanut, Cheyenne's brother was anxious for her to get down so that he could play with her, and she was squirming around in Barbara's arms and then in mine, before we finally said the hell with it and put her down on the floor. Frances came into the living room and we apologized for being so late in getting there. She said that when it got late, she didn't think that we were going to come down. She had been sick all week and had taken some over-the-counter medication similar to Nyquil

and gone to sleep. Elizabeth, who suffers from allergies and has sneezing attacks, had also taken some and that was why they didn't hear me when I had knocked on the door earlier in the evening.

I had a small problem. I didn't have enough gas in the van to take Michael and D.J. all the way back down to Peggy's and then get back to the gas station at Zion's Crossroads. The last thing we needed was to be stranded on the road in pouring down rain, so I had to find a gas station that was still open this late.

D.J. suggested that we go to a station across the Buckingham County Bridge called Jack's who was open, but we had only \a very few minutes to get there before they closed. Barbara was talking to Frances as we left, and drinking a cup of coffee. Elizabeth, still groggy and sleepy, was sitting on the sofa, and at first was uncommunicative, and then had a bit of an attitude for a few minutes, but soon settled down. I don't blame her a bit, though. If I was comfortable in my bed and sound asleep, only to be rudely waked up suddenly I would be grumpy too!

We made it to the station with just minutes to spare and got gas and drove back to Frances', where we found them talking about the trip and having a cup of coffee. I decided since I was tired and a little sleepy, it wouldn't be a bad idea to have a cup myself so I wouldn't risk falling asleep behind the wheel on the drive home. We stayed for about an hour or so before finally heading out. I was totally exhausted, having worked a full shift that day and here we were already into the day of the trip and I hadn't had the chance to close my eyes at all.

We drove the boys back to Peggy's, pulling into the driveway just long enough to let them get out and didn't bother to shut off the motor or anything. We backed out and headed home, blowing the horn as we pulled onto the highway. Barbara had Cheyenne wrapped in her blanket, and she reclined her seat for the ride, both of them settling down to at least get a little rest during the drive. I said a silent prayer that God be the one to guide the van as it traveled down the highway and to see us all safely home.

Destination: Columbus

The insistent buzzing of the alarm clock on my nightstand brought me abruptly out of a deep slumber, and I slowly opened one eye as I reached sleepily over to turn it off. I rolled over onto my back while stretching my arms above my head as I inched down farther under the covers against the chill of the air conditioned room. I definitely have not had nearly enough sleep I thought to myself as I slowly wiped the sleep from my tired eyes, and tossed back the cover to get out of bed. I made my way to the bathroom and then put on my pajamas as I walked toward the living room to wake Barbara, who was still asleep on the sofa. Shaking her slowly I told her it was time to get up as I walked into the kitchen for something cool to drink.

I often wondered how in the world she managed to sleep on the sofa night after night, but had to admit that it must be a lot more comfortable than the short loveseats we used to have back when I was first going through the treatments after having the PEG tube inserted in my stomach. She was afraid that sleeping with me during that time would cause problems if she accidentally touched it or it got tangled in her gown or something, and had begun sleeping in the living room for the time being. Afterwards, when we bought the new mattress, I made the mistake of buying an extra firm set and it was one that she could lay on for only short periods of time without pain in her back or hips.

As I used the bathroom and washed my face to wake myself even more, she went into the kitchen to start a pot of coffee. Figuring that our hot water heater as usual would have to build up before she could shower, I opted to go ahead and grab mine and take care of my other toiletries and get dressed before having coffee. We had not had the opportunity to do much in the way of getting everything together the day before and had a lot of small chores to finish before we left home and I knew her well enough by now to know that Barbara would finish everything that needed to be done before showering and getting dressed for the day.

Since we had located the carry on bag and the wheeled piece of luggage that we were going to be using for the trip the day before, we also took the time to look through the outfits that we had available and had chosen the ones each of us would pack. The first priority of the day after showering and dressing was to pack those and to be sure that we had everything else that would be essential in the luggage as well. Barbara, being a very resourceful and organized person had taken the time to make a list of needed items beforehand. It proved to be a very smart idea and if it had not been for the list we would have surely forgotten something that we would have needed once we were at the hotel. While I was getting dressed in our bedroom, she was gathering the notebooks, highlighter pens, pencils and her schoolbooks for Kaplan University, making sure that the Trac Fone was fully charged from the night before, and got it turned on and ready to use, packing the charger into the carry on bag.

As we sat down at he kitchen table to enjoy our cups of coffee we went over the list together in case there was something that she had somehow overlooked when she made the list, but she had done such a good job there was nothing that I could think to add to it. She had even remembered that I was running low on Oral Balance gel for dry mouth that I use at night before going to bed, and had gone to Wal-Mart to buy a tube, which they thankfully had in stock in the pharmacy. She had also picked up extra toothpaste and small plastic travel bottles to take a supply of shampoo, conditioner, body lotion and mouthwash with us. Neither of us liked the ones that are provided by the hotels and much preferred what we were used to using at home.

After finishing our coffee, we moved into the bedroom to begin packing the clothing and the essentials in the bag to be checked. We had been given good advice by seasoned travelers not to check the laptop computer when we got to the airport, and the manager at Rent-A-Center had put it into a backpack which would make it easy for me to carry. We used a large green canvas bag for our carry-on baggage, and of course Barbara had her purse to deal with. Having traveled to New York in 2006, we learned a lot of dos and don'ts about what airport security allowed in luggage. All liquids had to be less than 4 oz. and secured in a quart size zipper seal bag, with one allowed in carry-on luggage and another in the checked baggage.

Barbara's aunt, Annie May Maddox had offered to go with us to the airport, drop us off and then she would drive the van to her house in Howardsville until we were due back on Sunday evening, when she would drive to the airport and pick us up. I know it sounds like a confusing plan, but the whole point of it was to prevent us from having to pay a high fee for parking the van in the lot at the airport. Annie had never driven a van before and was leery of it but said that she was willing to try. However, as the time got closer to departure and she and Barbara talked about it, they both decided that it would be much better if we could find someone living close to us to give us a ride. It would save on driving time and gas expense.

The day before the trip, Annie was finally able to convince her brother James, who lived the next street over from the trailer park, to go with us instead. It did make a lot more sense, because he could ride with us and drive the van back to our house and park it and then slide over to his house, and reverse it when we landed on Sunday. Barbara had called him the night before to thank him and tell him that he didn't have to meet us at the house until 8 a.m. so that we would have time to get everything packed and ourselves ready. James had never driven into the airport and I had to make sure to show him the way to get in and out when we got there. It still confuses me and we've been there several times now, and used to do a lot of pick ups for the yard sales around that area of Earlysville. It seems like I miss the road to the terminal each and every time and have to turn around and go back.

The sun was shining very bright and the humidity was very noticeable in the air that early, so it promised to be another scorcher and we were glad that we were getting out of town before it hit. Our flight wasn't scheduled for departure until 11:15, although they usually board about 15 to 20 minutes prior to take off, so we still had plenty of time and there was no need to rush. I had forgotten to get matches (since we were not going to have a lighter) when I had stopped for gas, drinks and cigarettes at Sheetz on the way to the airport, and after I had unloaded our luggage and the wheelchair, James drove down to the little grocery store right off of the main highway to get us several books.

The Lance Armstrong Foundation had purchased our tickets electronically, so they were listed in the computer system. In order to secure our boarding passes we were to go to the ticket counter of US Air and show our drivers licenses to receive them. The ticket agent was very jovial and adept at his job, and he handed our boarding passes and had our luggage checked, along with a claim ticket for the wheelchair within just a matter of minutes. One of the regulations at the airport is that they do not allow any vehicle to park out front and be left unattended. James had returned with the matches while we were checking in, and he had left them with one of the security guards who gave them to us as we approached the restrooms.

It was still much too early to go through the check-in process, so after using the restrooms, we went outside the front entrance to talk, smoke a cigarette and finish our drink which we knew we wouldn't be allowed to carry with us during the check-in procedure. All of the cab drivers who were waiting for those who needed transportation and the guards were friendly and we chatted with them while we were outside. Finally, the heat became a little much and we decided to go on inside and get ready to board the flight when it was announced.

It was ironic that when we had returned from our trip to New York after attending the SPOHNC event in 2006, we both had made the statement that we weren't planning on flying again…Time and opportunity had definitely changed our minds about it, however. It might sound silly to some people who do it frequently until it becomes something of a habit. But for both Barbara and myself, who until we became involved with cancer and advocating for it after my diagnosis, had never flown before, it was a new adventure and something that we were looking forward to today.

The actual flight was fascinating, it was dealing with all of the regulations, stipulations and moving through the system that was totally frustrating and nerve wrecking.

As we entered the check-in area, a security guard asked for our boarding passes and drivers licenses again before allowing us to proceed any further. We sat the carry-on bag onto the conveyor belt, along with Barbara's purse and I had to remove the laptop from the backpack and place it into the tray separately, sending the backpack through the x-ray machine by itself. Next, Barbara had to remove her shoes (thankfully she had worn slip on ones that were easy to take off and put on), and I had to remove my belt, change from my pockets, the Trac Fone and anything else metal, along with my tennis shoes. Since Barbara was sitting in the wheelchair, they pushed her through the other side where they had a woman guard complete her check-in. They did a pat down, and checked the chair using a wand-type metal detector and we were then told which gate we would be boarding from, and made our way over to it.

The enticing aromas of the brewed coffee available at a station in the waiting area was very tempting for both of us, but we decided to pass on it because of the fact it caused both of us to go to the bathroom way too much, and the one thing that both of us wanted to do was to avoid having to use the lavatory on the airplane. There was a television in the waiting area tuned into CNN News and we listened to that for a while. We actually saw one of the headlines that said: "McCain stomping with Lance Armstrong in Ohio." We both smiled at that because one of the events for the Summit was a Town Hall Meeting with John McCain, scheduled for 6:30 that evening. I went down to the vending machines located on one end of the waiting room and got us a bag of chips each and a soda to share while we were waiting. Shortly after that, one of the ground crew came in to say that they would be pre-boarding us as soon as the plane arrived and had gone through the required maintenance check.

They were really nice and wanted to make boarding as easy for Barbara as possible and they brought out what is called an "aisle chair" that will go up the ramp to the plane, and is then guided between the row of seats, where she could simply slide into her assigned seat, and they worked efficiently and we were onboard with minimal fuss and effort. We were flying on one of the smaller planes just like we had for our first flight, and it was cramped with very little leg room and access to the seats. Barbara had the window seat but offered to switch with me. I wasn't sure if she was just being nice or if she really wanted to switch, but I declined the offer and remained where I was. The seatbelts did not have much flexing ability so she asked the flight attendant if he would bring her a set of extensions so that she could fasten her belt, and it seemed like he was distracted by everything going on around him. By the time he finally remembered to bring them, the pilot had started the engines and we were actually moving down the runway in preparation for take-off. This would be a short flight, averaging just shy of an hour before we landed. We were actually looking forward to some of the events that had been advertised for the Summit and all I was hoping for was the chance to rest for a while, the chance to freshen up and a nutritious snack before we had to attend any sort of function with a crowd of people.

LaGuardia Airport in New York had really been impressive by the size of the facility and the number of shops that were located inside, but it in no way prepared us for what greeted us as we entered Douglas airport in Charlotte! It seemed to stretch for miles on end, with shops galore, ranging from NASCAR memorabilia (after all it is the stockcar capitol), restaurants of all kinds, wine and sports bars, gift shops, fruit stands, bookstores, clothing outlets, phone centers—and they were just what we could see as we came inside. Reaching into the side pocket of the backpack, I took out our boarding passes to check the number of the gate we needed, and let out a long sigh. I had no idea where to find the gate, but I knew without a doubt that it meant I would be doing quite a lot of walking to find it.

The lack of sleep the night before was now taking it's toll on me and I was beginning to feel tired and cranky, not to mention parched and my stomach was protesting that it wanted food—and soon. Ok, I thought— first things first. I was going to find the gate that we would need, let them do their damned check-in procedure since it was a different airport, and then I was going in search of food and a nice cold beer if one could be found. It would probably be triple the price I paid for one in Virginia but by this point I really wasn't thinking about money. The signs overhead kept teasing us that our gate was straight ahead, and the more I walked the farther it seemed. I finally noticed that there were carts passengers were riding, being driven by employees of the airport, and finding one that was empty at the moment, I asked for help.

The driver, a tall slender black male was very friendly, and after checking our boarding passes for the gate we needed, helped Barbara onto the cart and then strapped the wheelchair onto the back along with the luggage, as I sat beside Barbara and we were off! Traveling through the throngs of people definitely took skill as some refused to make way for the driver to get around them, which I thought was rude, but I kept silent. The driver was nice enough to stop at the nearest restrooms so we wouldn't have to find them after check-in, and we were finally dropped at the proper desk and he wished us a safe trip before turning around and driving off from the direction we had come from. We waited our turn to complete the check-in and afterwards decided to get some fresh air and allow Barbara to smoke a cigarette and to call my mother to let her know that we had landed safely in Charlotte and was waiting for our connecting flight to Columbus. We had an hour's layover which was plenty of time to go outside and to get refreshments and a snack before we got on the plane again. One of the uniformed security guards told us where to go to find the smoking area, and after getting Barbara settled outside and leaving the bags for her to watch, I returned to the terminal in search of food and drink. It wouldn't take long to find either one with all of the choices to make—or would it?

I couldn't believe the way our luck was running today, but it evidently was going to stay true to form and do all it could to test our patience and flexibility to the limit. I was stopped by one of the guards and told that since I was reentering the building that I would have to go back through another check-in. What? You've got to be kidding me! I had to strip off my belt and everything else to just get a damn soda and snack? These people were absolutely amazing and unreal. I could understand the fact that it paid for them to be cautious, but this was a bit extreme, I remember grumbling to myself as I emptied my pockets one more time, taking off shoes and walking through the electronic monitoring system. I knew Barbara was probably wondering where the hell I had disappeared to, and couldn't wait to see her face when I told her and then reminded her that she would have to go through the same thing when she came back in. I knew she would be really pissed off, but what could we say? We would just have to grin and bear it.

By the time we drank the soda and smoke a cigarette, went back inside and made it through the damn check-in one more time, when we got to the boarding gate we discovered that we had missed the connecting flight we were supposed to be on, and had to stand there helplessly and wait until the man behind the counter managed to book us on the next flight leaving Charlotte for Columbus. Damn, damn, damn! That meant getting in even later, and we would either be pushing the time to the limit or maybe even miss out on attending the Town Hall meeting all together. We would still have to find our luggage, secure a taxi to the hotel and then complete the registration before getting to our room.

When they called our boarding for the flight, we were quite surprised that instead of flying on one of the small aircraft we had arrived on, we would instead be in a regional jet. Now I thought, this is more like it. The tunnel to the door of the plane was hot and humid with no air stirring whatsoever, and we were both sweating profusely by the time the aisle chair had gained the entryway to the plane. Looking around, there was plenty of leg room and the seats were very luxurious in appearance and I couldn't wait to sink into one and relax. I opened the luggage compartment overhead and put everything except Barbara's purse inside, and sat down at the same time that the stewardess brought Barbara the extender for the seatbelt. This was the style of plane that is often depicted in television shows and the movies I thought, smiling. We were going to be late arriving, but at least it was in style.

When the plane was in flight and had reached the proper altitude the stewardesses brought the drink cart around and served juices (or you could purchase a beer for $5) and a light snack for the passengers to enjoy during the flight, which was a nice surprise. I had to visit the lavatory as much as I was hoping to avoid it, and Barbara had ordered me a cranberry cocktail since there were not many juices available that I really enjoyed, taking a Coke for herself. I was relaxed finally and it seemed like we had just taken off from Charlotte when the pilot came on to announce that we were approaching Columbus and would be landing within 15 minutes. The speed that the jet could travel had actually cut the flying time listed in half.

After entering Port Columbus Airport we used the restrooms and then went to the baggage claim area to find our luggage. There were passengers waiting around the conveyor belt and children milling around, playing. It took almost three quarters of an hour before we were finally able to locate our bags and begin to make our way to the main entrance. We were going to be staying at the Hyatt on Capitol Square and unfortunately they did not provide shuttle service from the hotel. I would have to locate a cab to take us there, and had been warned it would cost approximately $20 for the fare.

Taxi drivers lined the street, each vying for the passengers to ride with them. The wheelchair was difficult to fit into the trunk of a regular car without a lot of hassle, so we located a driver who had a van which would be easier. He didn't take the time to secure the chair or the luggage when he loaded it into the back and it moved everywhere each time he had to brake for traffic or to stop at a light. We were very impressed with the hotel as he pulled up in front where valets in uniform waited to assist people in unloading and parking their vehicles. There was a LIVESTRONG banner around the column of the hotel welcoming people to the Summit, and a valet helped me unload our things. I paid the driver and he was trying to take off before I had the chance to retrieve the laptop, and I had to tell him to wait.

A black porter (his name we learned was James) had placed our luggage onto one of the luggage carriers and we followed him into the lobby of the hotel. We were both impressed with the luxury and set up of the lobby. The floor tiles gleamed and in various sitting areas, there were very nice suites of furniture sitting upon rich oriental area rugs, with plants on stands and magazines on the coffee tables. The front desk was deep dark cherry wood and gleamed from being polished, behind which stood the hotel assistant manager waiting to assist us with registration. He was very personable and friendly and within minutes we were checked in and had the key to our room, which we learned was on the 10th floor, and James was waiting with the elevator to take our luggage upstairs for us. He took the key (which resembled a credit card) and unlocked the door of the room, stepping back to allow me to push the wheelchair in first. After Barbara got out, I folded it up, placing it along the wall next to the bathroom until we needed it again.

James unloaded the luggage carrier, placing the bags on the luggage rack beside the television armoire/dresser combination standing on one wall (a desk with chair was on the other side), before taking the ice bucket provided by the hotel to the machine down the hall and filling it for us. The room was very spacious and well organized. The bed was a king size pillow top with lots of pillows (including decorative ones) and thick blankets. We were both tired by then and decided to see if it was going to be comfortable. As we both stretched out, James got a good chuckle from the huge sigh of contentment each of us released as our bodies seemed to sink down into the mattress like it was custom made for us. Before leaving, he told us to be sure to just call the front desk and ask for him personally if there was anything that he could do to help us during our stay. We thanked him and just lay on the bed for a few minutes.

Since we had missed our connecting flight from Charlotte and had to wait to take one later in the afternoon, we had arrived too late to attend the Town Hall meeting with John McCain, the Republican candidate for President. There was a "Welcome to the 2008 Summit" billboard displayed on an easel in the lobby, and beside it was a schedule of the events and the times of pickup/drop off and destinations for the events that would be held at different locations on the campus of Ohio State University. Instead of worrying about missing the event with McCain, after we rested and caught our breath, we took the time to unpack and put away our clothes. The outfits we would wear were hung in the closet, while under clothes, t-shirts and socks were put into the drawers underneath the television. We also unpacked the toiletries and put them in the bathroom for easy access, opting to leave the laptop and school books packed until Barbara was going to use them.

We hadn't had much to eat or drink during the entire trip and we were both feeling hunger pangs by then, so we went downstairs to the registration desk to inquire about places close by to eat dinner. After getting information on them, we headed in the direction given. Upstairs in the hotel was a shopping mall that was similar in size (and some of the shops) to that of Fashion Square Mall in Charlottesville. We decided to have dinner at a restaurant called San Francisco Oven which offered a variety of pasta dishes to choose from. We both ordered Chicken Parmesan that came with a side order of house salad and soft drink. I got the drink because it came with the meal (figuring that maybe Barbara would want it to go with her meal or for later) but chose a Budweiser for myself. We looked around the restaurant and chatted while we waited for our food. There was a rock 'n roll band playing outside on the patio, and although I've definitely heard better bands from the days when I used to frequent bars and nightclubs, it was something to at least listen to for a while. From the signs outside, it was a summer event that happened each and every Thursday evening, with different bands performing each week.

We sat there in companionable silence, enjoying the food which was absolutely delicious and just relaxing after a long and trying day of driving, flying and hustling from one place to the other. We had brought extra spending money with us but had made a pact to be careful what we spent it on so that we would have some left over when we got home. After we finished our dinner and used the bathroom, I went to the register and bought one more beer, and we decided to go outside on the patio for a while. It was also the smoking area for the hotel, although we noticed that some of the guests preferred to go across the street out from the front entrance.

Barbara, determined to get pictures during this trip to have for keepsakes and to share with our support group, had her digital camera with her in her purse, but I went up to the room and got the camera and bag that she had borrowed from Annie May just in case the memory card of the digital got full. As we sat there listening to the band and sipping our drinks, we noticed that the patio seemed to be turning into a gathering place for those delegates who had come to participate in the Summit that would begin in earnest the following morning. We had also arrived too late to attend the registration for the event that had been held at the State House directly across the street from the hotel. Barbara asked several people about when we could register and was told that we could do it before the opening session the following morning.

We were pleasantly surprised when Dan Waeger from the National Coalition for Cancer Survivorship greeted us while we were sitting there. We didn't know that he had planned on attending the Summit, although Anne Willis, one of the other staff members had said that she was planning on attending. It turned out that Dan, along with a co-worker and his fiancée had driven over 6 hours to attend the Town Hall meeting. Unfortunately, when they had arrived at their destination, the Secret Service people with John McCain had refused to allow them to go inside. It seemed that those people who were leaders in the Armstrong Army had received precedence over the other delegates attending. Dan, to say the least, was totally disappointed. He said that it had been the one event that he had definitely been looking forward to the most.

There was a little place called Darby's Café, (which was an extension of Darby's Sports Bar in the hotel itself) located on the patio and people were eating and drinking as they chatted and listened to the band, which played until around 9:30 before they began packing up their equipment to leave. We stayed outside until around 11, when we both began to fight exhaustion and decided to call it a night, heading inside to the comfortable bed for what we hoped was a good night's sleep.

THE SUMMIT BEGINS

Our day began bright and early at 5 a.m. when the front desk delivered the wake up call that Barbara had requested before turning out the lights the night before. We had to be dressed and downstairs for pick up by the buses heading to the Summit by 6:30, and the last thing we wanted to do was rush in order to be ready. The bed was so comfortable that I slept like a baby, and didn't want to get up when Barbara shook me awake. I wasn't still tired but it just felt so good to lay in a comfortable bed for a change. Humph! It must have been comfortable because I woke up in the same position I went to sleep in, evidently not moving a muscle all night long.

I went into the bathroom to shower while Barbara got out the clothes that we would wear for the day, and organized pens and paper to take any notes of interest during the sessions. It took me a few minutes to figure out how to adjust the water temperature to a comfortable level before stepping under the spray. I didn't particularly like the shower because it was a handicapped accessible one and to me it didn't put out the pressure of a normal shower head, but I made the best of it. I had to admit that the hotel had been very accommodating for those who suffered disabilities. There were handrails in the shower and beside the commode, the sink was lower for easy access and the room had wide doorways for wheelchairs or walkers.

After showering and cleaning my dentures, I came into the bedroom to get dressed. I didn't know if anyone was a NASCAR fan but I chose to wear my black Dale Earnhardt, Sr. t-shirt (and of course I was wearing #3 on my hat) with jeans and tennis shoes. I thought that perhaps the weather would be too hot here in Columbus for my black suede boots and it definitely wouldn't help my feet having to do a lot of walking and pushing the wheelchair, either.

After Barbara had finished her shower and gotten dressed, we made sure that we had the room key and everything else that we might need for the day before heading downstairs and making our way to the bus stop. There were already several ladies there that we introduced ourselves to and we spent a few minutes getting acquainted while waiting for the bus to arrive. I had to load the wheelchair on the bus, and one of the ladies helped me fold it up because Barbara chose to sit on one of the seats instead of the chair. I was glad, because I wasn't sure how the chair would respond if the driver had to stop suddenly or turned a sharp corner.

As we approached the campus of Ohio State University, I could hardly believe it. I have followed sports and college football enough over the years to realize that this school could boast about having one of the best records in Ivy League play, and here I was about to step onto their hallowed campus for the first time. Except for attending basketball games at John Paul Jones Arena for the University of Virginia back home, this was the first time I had been on another University campus and it was exciting.

We didn't know where we were to go to do the registration for the event, so after unloading the wheelchair from the bus and getting Barbara settled into it with her purse and notebooks, I began following the others who were making their way around the sidewalks of the campus. It was a bit chilly this morning, but the sun was slowly rising on the horizon and it promised to be another warm but hopefully less humid day than what we had experienced in Virginia. The lawns were well maintained with an abundance of trees and shrubbery planted along the walkways, and flowers in various containers closer to the buildings.

We entered a large building which we learned later was called Mershon Auditorium. Once inside, Barbara needed to use the restroom and afterwards, we made our way down the lobby to where there were several tables set up and manned by volunteer staff members for the event. The first order of business was to give our names to receive our registration packet (which included name tags and an itinerary, a LAF tee-shirt and tote bag each. Barbara, always thinking about resources she could use to help others, went to a table that had information about the Foundation and began talking to one of the staff members. She collected a guide to all Legislators for Congress, and filled out a card to become a leader in the Armstrong Army.

Shortly afterwards, it was time to enter the auditorium itself for the opening ceremonies of the Summit. One of the volunteers who was working the doorway lead us to another farther down that was for those delegates with assistive devices. We weren't as close to the stage as either of us would have preferred, being up on a balcony and having to watch the speakers via large screened television. Lance Armstrong opened the ceremony telling a few jokes that brought laughter from those in the audience about his dancing skills compared to cycling which he knew about. The President and CEO of Ohio State University welcomed everyone to his institution and wished each attendee success over the weekend.

The keynote speaker for this morning's session was Dr. Richard Carmona, the 17th Surgeon General of the United States. He served in office between 2002 and 2006, and shared his personal story about highlights from his career, and his involvement with cancer and LAF and the efforts it would require to make cancer a national priority. Having retired from his prestigious position in no way had any bearings on his determination to continue working to improve the health of Americans and his dedication to advancing treatments to conquer the insidious disease that affects 1 in 2 men and 1 in 3 women in America today.

The Foundation had set up huge tents outside of Mershon Auditorium to provide meals for those attending the events as well as the buildings spread out across the campus where different training tracks would occur. After closing the morning's general session, everyone filed out of the auditorium and began making their way back to the tent for a Continental Breakfast. I found a table where Barbara could easily access and get out of the wheelchair for a while, and after folding it so that it wouldn't be in other people's way, I went to get food for both of us. I would much rather have had something hot (like bacon and eggs with toast) but this would have to suffice until lunch time. At least my stomach wouldn't be rumbling while I was concentrating on at the training session.

After finishing breakfast we were to meet at the bus stop where the Foundation had contracted with the Columbus transit system to provide transportation to the buildings around campus where the Break out Tracks (training sessions) would be held during the day. Barbara and I had signed up for advocacy training and ours was at the Meiling Building. I became really frustrated when Barbara chose to walk onto the bus because the chair lift was not working and I had to struggle to get the chair onto the bus, and with so many people, it kept rolling and bumping into people. I could see right away that the transit system was in no way prepared to accommodate people with physical disabilities, which meant this was definitely going to be a nightmarish weekend as far as attending all of the sessions was concerned.

When we entered the Meiling Building, there were signs pointing to the two different training events being housed there for the weekend, and finding the one for advocacy 1, a LAF volunteer gave us directions on how to find the handicapped accessible entrance to the auditorium, which was located downstairs. We found it after getting turned around once, and as we entered the room it was huge, with tables set in rows like a basketball gymnasium and the padded chairs that swiveled, allowing the student to seat themselves. We folded Barbara's chair and put it in a corner to be out of traffic and took a seat at the first set of tables near the floor.

During the morning session, the speakers gave pointers on how to advocate at the different levels of Government, which having already been to Capitol Hill was not new to us, but it was good to hear how they perceived making a good impression on elected officials. However, we could not agree with some of the things they suggested, having learned first hand what did and did not work on the Washington political scene as far as gaining the attention of members of Congress. Perhaps it was because different organizations had different ways of approaching the same problem, and what worked for one did or did not work for the other. The second exercise on the agenda promised to be a little more interesting.

The leaders of the group divided all of those attending the session into groups of nine people, giving each group a name of an animal and once everyone had moved into their prospective groups, handed out digital cameras. Each group was to make a commercial explaining why cancer should be made a national priority, and each commercial would be judged on its merit, content and presentation after lunch, and the winner of the contest would be announced to the group. I participated with our assigned group, but for the life of me didn't see where they had said anything new or innovative that had not already been said a million times over. Well, so much for that, I thought. Surely another of the groups would definitely come up with something far better and win the contest.

As we sat on the patio having lunch a bit later, I could tell by the expression on Barbara's face that she had about reached the limit of her tolerance with the way the day was shaping up. I couldn't agree more and was disappointed in what I had experienced with "training" so far. The hot sun was making perspiration run down my back and my shirt had begun sticking to my skin which was very uncomfortable. After we finished lunch, we found a quiet, shady spot away from the food tent to cool off so Barbara could have a cigarette and call Frances to check on how Cheyenne was doing without us. Just as we had both feared, she was moody and not eating like she should and it caused a few tears to come to Barbara's eyes. We had definitely become attached to her in such a short time and she had us both wrapped around all 4 of her little paws. It didn't take long after that call to Frances for Barbara to decide that she was not going to spend the rest of the day sitting in that auditorium.

After returning for a few minutes, we left and had one of the LAF staff members who worked there call and arrange for someone from transit to pick us up to return us to the hotel. It sure sounded like a winner to me! They sent a handicapped accessible van this time to offer a ride for which we were grateful. Like Jaunt in Virginia, these were equipped with a motorized wheelchair lift which would keep me from straining muscles to load it myself. The driver wasn't accustomed to where to drop us off and at first, he was going to unload us at the back of the hotel which meant pushing her down the steep sidewalk to the front of the hotel to get inside. I was finally able to get him to pull up directly in front, but of course that didn't work out too well. He pulled the van too close to the sidewalk and didn't allow enough room for the lift to unload the chair, which damaged the armrest of it, and Barbara had to step out of the chair, have me unload it from the lift and then sit back down. Whew! Where did these people get their license, I wondered as I wheeled her inside the air conditioned lobby, which felt absolutely wonderful as it cooled our hot sweaty bodies down to a tolerable level.

The lobby of the hotel was fairly empty this time of the day, although there were clerks behind the registration desk who acknowledged us as we made our way to the elevator on the way to the room. It didn't take me long before I was stripping off the wet t-shirt and taking a cool shower to feel refreshed, and Barbara quickly shed her clothes and stepped into a warm bath and did her hair. We felt human and ready for something to snack on and a cool drink. The lady who was working the food tent had been gracious enough to provide us each with two sandwiches, fruit, snacks and sodas that we could have later for dinner.

We sat outside in the Courtyard for quite a while off and on during the afternoon and evening, and met quite a few of our fellow delegates who came in at different intervals from the training sessions. We made quite a few acquaintances and exchanged contact information with a few of them so that we could keep in touch. We took several pictures around the hotel: statues, the hotel lobby, signs for the event, some of the hotel personnel, and of course the water fountains in different areas of the complex.

We retired fairly early that night and enjoyed our dinner in the room, watching television while relaxing in bed. It was cool with the air conditioning running and it didn't take long before fell asleep while Barbara was still watching television, and eventually, she dozed as well. I woke her around 11 and she turned off the set, called the front desk to request the wake up call for 5 a.m. and it was lights out once again.

The next morning was a repeat of Friday, and by 10 a.m., we had discovered that it definitely wasn't going to be anything that we could gain from the conference that would be useful to us as far as how to advocate for better quality cancer care for Americans stricken with the disease, and we arranged for and received transportation back to the hotel before lunch, along with several snacks for the afternoon. I had been on a partial tour of the mall upstairs in the complex but Barbara had not. That was about to change today, which was our last full day in Columbus before flying home the following afternoon.

The mall was indeed very spacious and covered two floors of the complex, although we only took the time to tour the first level. There were numerous eating establishments, ranging from fast food and burgers, to barbeque, pizza and other pasta specialties, and several ice cream parlors. You could buy luggage and handbags, have shoes repaired, buy a gift of jewelry or flowers, pick up toys in a dollar place, or buy reading materials, just from the ones that we visited or walked by. The one that caught Barbara's immediate attention was Waldenbooks, which is one of the bookstores that we have in Virginia. I could see the wheels literally turning in her head as she asked me to push her inside and help her locate a manager. I knew instinctively what she was after: to find out how to market our book once it was published. I told you she was organized and resourceful, didn't I?

After maneuvering the chair close to the checkout and finding a cashier, she asked to speak with a manager and found out that the clerk was actually the assistant manager of the store, which was the next best thing. She explained that I, as a survivor of head and neck cancer, had written a book that was due to be published later this year, (hopefully before the holidays) and was wondering how we could get Waldenbooks to display our book in their stores. She congratulated us on the fact that we were going to be published and said that she would be glad to help us with any questions.

She explained that the best way to get an agreement established with the store was to approach the manager with a copy of the book in hand, and to request they agree to host a book signing. Her other suggestion was to tell everyone we know who is interested in buying a copy of the book to wait until the day of the signing to come to the store and buy the book while we were there. It would allow the personnel of the store to see just how popular the book would be, and would help nudge them toward ordering a larger quantity from the publisher. She also gave us a business card and asked that we send her a copy of the book when it was released and she would display it in the store there. It was nice to see that there was a local author from Publish America with one of her books displayed near the cash register. We left the store feeling very good about the prospect of working with Waldenbooks by home in Virginia.

We turned in fairly early that night since the following day would be quite a hectic one, with the closing ceremonies for the Summit, having to pack and the hustle and bustle of reaching the airport and flying home, which would require another layover in Charlotte before finally returning to Virginia later in the evening.

Return to Virginia

We decided when we retired to our room for the evening that we were not going to ask for a wake-up call the following morning, and would skip out on attending the closing ceremonies. The staff of the hotel had been gracious enough to extend the check-out time until one in the afternoon since the event didn't close until noon. However, most people who were actually going to the ceremony would take their luggage with them and store it in a space that was being set aside for that purpose. After the ceremony, the buses providing transportation would then take them directly to the airport for their flights home.

I think that by this time both Barbara and I had dealt with lugging and transporting the wheelchair all we were capable of doing, and so we decided to sleep in for a while and then take our time in packing for the return home, so that we wouldn't run the risk of leaving something important behind. While I took a shower, Barbara began organizing our belongings to be packed, and the first thing she did was to pack everything that would be allowed in the carry-on bag, trying to pack it neat so that nothing that could be damaged would shift while in transport. Having had to deal with both the backpack and the carry-on during the flight in to Ohio, we decided that the best thing would be to just check both bags—one as hers and one as mine. Then I would handle the computer while all she had was her purse. It sure sounded good to me. The less I had to be responsible for the better; maybe I would reach home without feeling totally exhausted.

After our showers we both felt refreshed and ready to face the long day ahead. Before she got dressed in what she was wearing home, Barbara went through and packed everything so that we were ready to leave. After dressing, she called down to the registration desk and asked the clerk to inform James that we were ready to check out of the room so that he could take our baggage downstairs and we could turn in the room key. We weren't going to spend any more time in the room and it would give the housekeeping staff an ample amount of time to clean it for the next guest who would check in.

Within several minutes of calling the desk, James, in full uniform with a jovial and friendly smile on his face, knocked softly on the door to announce his arrival. As he loaded our two bags on his cart, he asked about our stay and we told him that we had enjoyed it very much and asked if there was somewhere we could get a nice strong cup of hot coffee without spending a fortune for it, since by this time our money was slowly dwindling down and we needed some for gas to be able to pick Cheyenne up once we landed in Charlottesville. I explained to him that we were going to go outside to the courtyard for a little while, and he said that he would let me know when he had the coffee ready. Several minutes went by, and true to his word, we each had a large cup of deliciously aromatic coffee in front of us.

I left for a few minutes to use the bathroom and when I came back, Barbara was having a very animated discussion with another woman, who it turned out had also been a scholarship delegate to the Summit, who had opted to skip out on the closing ceremonies. She had already checked out of the hotel and had a carry-on bag sitting in the chair next to her. We sat around talking and getting to know each other for a couple of hours, killing time before leaving for the airport.

Her name was Andra Baker and she was from Texas, and lived in a suburb of Dallas called De Soto. She bought refreshments for us and we chatted about our diagnoses, treatments, and some of the advocacy work we had each done, and just sharing experiences of all types. The hotel had been gracious enough to give us a voucher to pay for the taxi which would take us back to the airport, so we offered to let her ride with us which would save her cab fare. It was the least that we could do because we had really enjoyed her company, and we had exchanged contact information to keep in touch with each other.

I excused myself just shy of the check-out time and had the clerk at the front desk call for a taxi for us and we went inside to tell James that we were ready to leave. When the taxi arrived, the driver helped to store the chair and luggage in the back and we were on our way. The driver didn't seem to happy that he would be getting a voucher instead of cash, and we spent a good deal of the time on the ride trying to convince him to return to the hotel with the information on the voucher filled out so that he would be paid. Barbara and I were the first to get out of the cab, so we do not know if he did or did not return to the hotel.

We had learned a hard lesson in Charlotte when we missed our connecting flight so this time after going through check-in and locating the gate from which we would be departing, except for quick trips to the restrooms, we stayed put until it was time to board the plane. The loud speaker informed passengers of delayed and cancelled flights all afternoon because of inclement weather across the country. Thankfully, ours would be the one flight that would depart on schedule, and we were both really looking forward to getting home. We flew from Columbus to

Charlotte via the regional jet like we had arrived on, and once again depended on the motorized car to navigate the airport. Our flight to Charlottesville left on time and we arrived just after seven in the evening.

We had been unable to get an answer when we tried to call James the entire day, and just assumed that he would remember what time our plane was supposed to land so that we wouldn't have to wait for him to pick us up outside the airport. After retrieving our luggage, which took just a minimum amount of time, we went outside in search of our van. We were totally shocked to see his wife and the rest of the family instead of James. We found out that the reason was simple: James had suffered another slight heart attack that morning and had been admitted to University of Virginia Medical Center for observation. I know that it upset Barbara because she worries about everybody and is always calling him to see how he is feeling and if there is anything that she can do to help him.

Nancy (his wife) was driving their van, which is an exact replica of ours. She said that she didn't like driving other people's vehicles and that is why she brought theirs. We chatted about small things during the ride home, and we thanked them as I unloaded the bags and the wheelchair. I know that Barbara, while glad to be home, was thinking about Cheyenne, and was anxious to get down to Frances' to pick her up. It wasn't that we doubted that Frances and Elizabeth would take good care of her, but we were worried that she was still slacking back on eating and we had missed her more than we thought we would.

I put the wheelchair on the back deck and then thought better of it, and took it inside and left it sitting in the kitchen, putting the baggage in the bedroom, used the bathroom and locked the door behind me. I had unlocked our van before going inside and Barbara was already sitting inside, with the window down and her seatbelt fastened, ready to go. I stopped at D's Market on Route 33 and put gas in the van and bought us something to drink before heading to Fluvanna.

We arrived just after 9 and Frances must have been expecting us, because before I had the chance to turn the lights and motor off, the outside light flicked on, and Elizabeth stuck her head outside, telling us to come on inside. Almost as soon as we entered the door, Cheyenne was whimpering, jumping up on us, with her tail wagging 90 miles an hour! Think she missed us? As Barbara sat down, Cheyenne jumped from the floor onto her chest, whimpering and whining and licking her face, neck and hands nonstop. When I picked her up she repeated all of it with me and then didn't want to be put down on the floor. So I sat down in the wooden rocker and held her, with her laying her head on my arm and promptly taking a power nap.

Frances made some coffee and we had a cup with her, telling about the events of the trip and just visiting for a little while. It turned out we stayed way longer than either of us had planned on doing, and when we finally glanced at the clock sitting on a bookshelf, we were shocked to see that it was well after midnight. Yikes! I had to get up in a few hours because I was scheduled to return to work at 7 the next (uh, this) morning. I knew I would no more than lay my head on the pillow, fall asleep and then be shaken awake by the buzzing of that infernal alarm clock. Oh well, I would definitely be ready to go straight to bed when I got home that afternoon. But all in all, the opportunity of attending the 2008 Summit had been worth the frustration, hustle and bustle, and the traveling. And, yes—it was even worth the sleep that I had missed out on getting. While I love adventure, I was definitely ready for some quality down time to rest and let life return to normal for at least a little while before we were in the midst of another one.

Survival Tips

Barbara and I kept a list of some of the things that helped us on our journey through cancer and I would like to share them with you. Please note that while these tips will not apply to everyone diagnosed with cancer, you may find something that will help in certain areas or it may be that perhaps you know someone who has been searching for this information that you share with them.

Carry a pocket-size calendar with you at all times. It is a great way to keep track of appointments, and a referral for doing interviews, your story, or filling out applications, etc.

Contact the Lance Armstrong Foundation at www.livestrong.org for a copy of the Livestrong Survivor's notebook. It contains inspirational stories of cancer survivors, resources and is a great way to document tests, treatments, surgeries and other pertinent information, and most of it's FREE!!!!

If you prefer, ask your doctor or clinical social worker to print out copies of your records and keep them in a personal file folder by the dates.

Whenever you are referred to a new doctor and/or clinic, be sure to tell them that you are a cancer survivor, and ask them if they are experienced in treating those who have had cancer.

If you are uncertain about a specific test that a physician other than your oncologist, chemotherapy physician and/or surgeon orders, ask your cancer team if it is appropriate and safe to have it done.

If you are having trouble obtaining an appointment for a clinic (ex: eye clinic) then call your cancer doctor or their nurse. Often times, they can get you an expedited appointment.

Keep a Journal. This is your personal space, written by you in any way you choose. It is a way to record things such as feelings, symptoms, side effects, medications, concerns or events. It is a way for you to let go—put into words feelings of negativity that can hamper your progress; but also a wonderful way to record special milestones of your journey to recovery.

It is ok to cry. Tears are a way to relieve built up tension and stress. Just don't stay in that mode.

Keep the weekends light. There is nothing about cancer and the stress of appointments and other related business of the disease that will not keep until Monday. Concentrate on things you enjoy: a hobby, a book, movies, etc., to relax and let go.

Laughter is the best medicine. It can go a long way in helping you deal with day-to-day life.

Find a support group in your area that will give you the chance to talk to other survivors. They are often experienced in dealing with situations you may find yourself facing and can offer tidbits of how to deal with the problem.

Sometimes you may not feel like talking when people call. That's ok. Use your voicemail to record an update on your treatments, how you feel and that you will talk another time. Don't feel like you have to talk and repeat yourself.

Don't hesitate to ask for help. Grocery shopping, childcare, pet care, transportation to and from appointments, or just a "visit". Let family members and friends know what will help. They're often wondering what they can do to help you.

Those who experiences dry mouth and don't want to spend a lot of money on OTC products; some survivors prefer to use Extra Virgin Olive Oil as a way to cope with it, especially at night.

Another tip that they all share is to use room temperature water to wash down food at mealtime. Hot liquids irritate and cold (in ice) liquids constrict the throat—making swallowing more difficult.

Check with your cancer center to see if they have an Integrative Medicine Program. Massage therapy is a great "treat" for cancer patients—physically, emotionally and mentally. When you feel good physically, the rest follows.

Exercise as a way to relieve stress and to keep muscles loose and your body in shape. Simple things like taking a walk, stretching or yoga can be beneficial.

Save all receipts (ex: gas-to-and-from treatments, all prescription and over the counter products). They can be turned into your local Department of Social Services when you are applying for Medicaid and when you are due for a review of your case.

If you are enrolled in Medicare Part D and have products you use on a regular basis suggested to you by your physician, ask if they will be covered under the plan with a written letter from your physician. It is possible if they are key to your recovery or needed as part of the treatment for side effects.

The Patient Advocate Foundation is a wonderful resource. They may be helpful in finding financial resources for medical devices. They can be contacted at 1-800-532-5274 or www.patientadvocate.org.

Check with your local Ruritan Club. They sometimes have funds to help those in need with things such as medications or co-pays, especially with a letter of introduction and an outline of the need from the Patient Advocate Foundation.

NeedyMeds—This website lists medications available from pharmaceutical companies. You need your doctor, social worker or nurse to make the contact on your behalf.

For products pertaining to your recovery (for example dry mouth products, aspirin, etc) shop at Wal-Mart or Target instead of CVS or other drug stores. They have better pricing and you can ask them to stock the product or call ahead to make sure they order it for availability for when you wish to pick it up.

Contact area churches for special needs such as gas for transportation to and from treatments, special food needs, and help with shopping.

Call your local United Way Chapter for resource referrals in your area.

Apply for fuel assistance with your local Department of Social Services.

Contact your electric company and ask if they have budget billing. If so—sign up for it.

For Ensure and other nutritional supplements check with your oncology/radiology clinic or cancer center.

Ask the Clinical Social Worker if there are any special funds available for emergency assistance.

Cancer Care offers financial assistance for those going through treatments and also for those out of treatments. If eligible, these are provided through a grant provided by the Lance Armstrong

Foundation. For an application or to apply on-line visit www.cancercare.org.

Contact your local Department of Social Services to sign up for programs you may be eligible for: Food Stamps, General Relief, Home-Health Aides and Fuel Assistance.

Ask area businesses in your community to donate counter space for you to display a "donation jar". They are simple to make. Use a Mason or mayonnaise jar that is clean and lint-free; make a sign for the jar that includes a small picture, your name, what it will be used for (all donations to help with utility and medical expenses) and thank them (Your help is greatly appreciated. God Bless you). Next, using a wide blade kitchen knife cut a slot in the lid wide and long enough for folded bills and quarters to slide through easily. Make arrangements to check the jars once per week and set a time.

Hold Benefit Yard Sales-ask family members, co-workers, friends and neighbors from their garages or attics. Also advertise in a local free "ad taker" publication for usable household items for a benefit cancer yard sale. You'll be surprised at the response.

If you are denied Social Security Disability Benefits don't give up. Contact an attorney in your area who specializes in disability claims and who only gets paid if he wins. On average, he can push the appeal through fairly quickly; if it is not going to be fast enough, be sure to contact the Congressman for your district who will be able to assist you.

Check with your city or county office where you pay your taxes. Some localities offer tax or rent relief for persons on disability.

If and/or when you feel up to returning to work, talk with your cancer team to find out if they think you are physically up to the challenge, and explore all possibilities first.

Seek employment that is not as physically challenging. If you have special needs (ex: use a can to walk, have to have liquid hydration at all times) be sure to tell potential employers at the interview. Have a note from your physician to back up your statement.

Take frequent breaks for quick snacks like peanut butter crackers and Ensure for energy and calories.

Make copies of your paychecks and stubs for your records. Be sure to turn all pay stubs into your local Social Security Office, especially if you are on the 9-month "trial" work period.

If you have a computer, sign up for "online banking." It allows you to control your ability to pay your bills at your pace without leaving home. Most bills can be paid by using this method, and you can also sign up for email alerts from your bank.

Check out the classified section of your local newspaper or any free ad taker publications for needed items/services. They are often free or at reduced-cost. You can also place "wanted" ads in these for things you are in need of.

Use "junk" mail for writing grocery, to-do lists and other notes.

For ice: use soda bottles (2 Liter) that have been washed and filled with water and place in your freezer. It can be broken with a hammer for small ice when needed.

Keep all receipts for items pertaining to your treatment and/or recovery. These may be useful if you file Income Tax Returns. We use legal sized manila envelope to store ours.

Check with your local chapter of the American Cancer Society. They often time will help with gas vouchers for people in active treatment.

Invest in a good food chopper, blender and/or food processor. Most foods can be ground, chopped or pureed for easier swallowing and digestion.

Use Carnation Instant Breakfast or equivalent mixed with whole milk, fruit and vanilla ice cream in place of Ensure. Just as nutritious.

If you are having trouble with changes in your taste buds or would like to try new recipes, there is help available. SPOHNC has a wonderful cookbook called Eat Well, Stay Nourished: A Recipe and Resource Guide for Coping with Eating Challenges. SPOHNC can be reached at P.O. Box 53 Locust Valley, NY 11560, or www.spohnc.org or by calling 1-800-377-0928.

Call your local bread store (such as Flowers Baking Company). They give away day-old bread which is a good way to stock up because it can be frozen and taken out an hour or so before needed.

Check with your grocery store to see if they offer a savings card for items they put on sale/discount. It is a great way to stock up and save money at the same time.

Use local Food Banks and satellite food pantries for canned and dry goods. Some offer free home delivery if you are unable to drive

If you are a coffee drinker: save money by buying a permanent "mesh" coffee filter. It can be washed and reused, and is easily cleaned by adding 1 TBSP of bleach to dish water once a week. (Also a good way to keep your pot and basket stain-free).

For a fresh feeling mouth without the burn of alcohol, try Tom's alcohol-free mouthwash available at Wal-Mart. It has a cool crisp mint taste.

Clip coupons for your most used items. They also help stretch your Food Stamps.

Before beginning treatment, consult with a registered dietician in your cancer center. She will be a valuable partner to maintain proper nutrition and weight.

Eat frequent small snacks instead of large meals. Use "nutrient dense" foods like margarine, peanut butter, or mayonnaise as often as possible.

Prepare casseroles on your "good" days so you won't worry about mealtime. They can be easily defrosted in the microwave, or put into the oven an hour or so before meal time.

A wonderful resource for any patient (or caregiver) to have is called the Cancer Survival Toolbox from National Coalition for Cancer Survivorship. It is free for the asking and is an audio resource program, complete with guide book. Contact them at www.canceradvococacy.org or at 1-888-650-9127.

EPILOGUE

Be sure to get all of the information you can find to help you make well informed decisions about your course of treatment. But a word of caution: be careful where you get your information. Not all of it is legitimate, and it can be misleading and will only cause more confusion and aggravation.

Depend only on reputable organizations whenever possible. The internet can be good and bad. Use reliable sources such the National Coalition for Cancer Survivorship, The National Cancer Institute, and the American Cancer Society just to name a few.

Be involved in your treatment and care plan. Talk to your doctors- whether it is the Radiologist/Oncologist, the Surgeon or even other key members of the team. Don't be afraid to talk to them. They are there to help you, and the best way they can do that is if they know you are on the same page as they are.

Ask questions about your treatment: why each stage of it is important. Ask what the benefits are as far as your cancer, and what possible side effects you could experience as a result of the treatment. If you don't understand something they tell you, ask them to repeat it in another way that you can understand. Then, repeat it back to them so they know you understand.

If you think you will forget something, ask if you can record the visit, or if they will allow a friend or a family member to ask questions and take notes.

Associate with others will be your "support" mechanisms. That could be a spouse; a son or daughter, a close family friend, a Pastor or perhaps you are involved in a support group. It pays to have "somebody" you can turn to when you're feeling down or just need someone "there."

Turn negative into positive. I know you are probably thinking: what in the world can be positive about having cancer and dealing with all of these treatments, appointments and everything else that has happened because of it.

Well, there are positive things that happen as a result of you facing this disease. Perhaps it has brought you and the family closer together. Maybe someone you drifted apart in friendship with has come has come back into your life.

For myself and Barbara there were a lot of positive things, although at the time I guess we couldn't see them because we were so consumed with the treatments, etc. But now, looking after the fact, we had a lot going on that was good.

We met a lot of nice people who had already been where we were and could give us hints about how to survive it, and how to find something to hold on to when life seemed out to get us.

There were a lot of other things, too. We prayed together, which is something I'm sad to say we hadn't done a whole lot of before. So it was a good thing. It brought us closer together with God, and with our Faith. I can tell you that if it hadn't been for Him, we wouldn't have gotten through all of the medical, emotional, financial and just day-to-day problems we faced.

Advocate for yourself and others. I know, you're probably wondering what the hell advocacy is. You have no idea what it is or how to go about doing it. Well, I can tell you that you would be wrong.

You've actually done it all of your life and never realized it. That's right, you have! You've told your doctor you needed medication when you were sick. You've told employees when you needed a project finished.

Advocacy is standing up for what you believe in but also in something you need. So, we go through life advocating without ever really knowing that we do it.

When you advocate for others, you simply just expand what you've already been doing. For example, Barbara advocated on behalf of me with Social Services and all of the other organizations that I needed services from all through my cancer treatments.

And now that I am a "survivor", we've both broadened that perspective. Although we still do have to advocate for things that we need personally, we've become national advocates. We are working hard to push legislation through Congress which would benefit not only Dwayne in his survivorship status, but would also provide quality cancer for those now receiving treatment, and for those who will be diagnosed in the future.

It is a movement which has become very dear to us and one that we will continue working on for as long as cancer is the chronic, debilitating and life-altering disease that it is.

Share your story and experiences with people. By giving a little of yourself to those who are not aware of how cancer has affected you, it gives them a hands-on look at what it is like to deal with multiple treatments, how you handle the harsh reality of radiation, chemotherapy, constant doctor appointments, all of the things that you faced—and came through.

It gives them a better understanding, not only about how cancer is treated, but they understand YOU better. your grit, determination, your desire to come out on top, and how you take a practical approach—knowing what you need to do and doing it.

Most of all live each day to the full potential you possess. Make the most of every minute you have. Do the things you enjoy. Go to the places you love, and spend quality time enjoying life.

We defeat cancer when we don't allow it to change "US", who we really are on the inside. It can and will, change any and everything it touches on the outside. Don't allow to touch and change your dignity, your spirit, your faith.

They will be tested, make no mistake about that—and it will be time and time again on this journey. You can't stop that. But you can stop not allowing them to bend or break.

Don't forget to laugh, because sometimes it's the best medicine there is. I'm not saying that cancer, the treatment or anything else related to this debilitating disease is funny. But we can't be serious 24/7, without something to break the monotony of doctor appointments, tests and the challenges we face day to day.

As I was sitting at my computer writing this down and recalling what I went through, some of it was absolutely hilarious. The way I judged my surgeon in his funny little hat, or watching a comedy on television to relieve the tension and the pent up feelings of anger and frustration, now actually seems so funny I can still smile.

As I said in the hints section: WRITE, WRITE, and WRITE. Get a good sized college ruled notebook. Write an entry a day—what you feel, what you think, what made you smile, what made you cry—

whatever YOU want to write. Use it to vent your feelings. Use it to say hey I made it through ANOTHER day!

Don't be afraid to ask questions, questions and more questions. It will help your healthcare team stay on track, make them aware of where you are emotionally and physically, and let them know how you feel about the different levels of your treatment. Remember the saying—the only stupid question is the one you forgot to ask.

I feel that I have been truly blessed throughout this very difficult journey that I've been traveling for the past few years.

I received my treatment at an NCI (National Cancer Institute) Designated Facility, and I had a wonderful team of doctors, nurses and team members who made sure all of my needs were met.

However, it was my wife who was my lifeline on this journey. Her sheer will and determination make sure that I received good care and that I had the proper nutrition, and by keeping all of my appointments and my medications on schedule was amazing.

She refused to let me dwell on negative thoughts, and was always pointing out how far I had come and the positive things that were going on in my life and my treatment. There were times when food was the last thing I wanted, but she pushed and prodded until I ate.

When other health concerns developed, if she couldn't get a positive response from the clinic she was talking to, she never once hesitated to contact either my social worker or the nurse in my doctor's office to intervene on my behalf. But it was my faith in God that brought me through the darkest hours of the journey. I feel as if my cancer was a test for me to come through and that He isn't finished with me yet. I believe that He has a plan for me to follow while I'm here on earth.

It wasn't until after my wife and I became involved in with working with the national advocacy groups and we learned how much of an impact cancer has on people's lives, and that our healthcare system is not as equipped to handle cancer patients and survivors' needs as it should be, that I realized how I could use my journey through cancer as a teaching tool and stepping stone to help others.

As a survivor, I can use what we learned on a personal level and by utilizing the media, newspapers, magazines, and internet or by speaking to groups of people, I can make a difference.

I can also lobby my elected officials at the local, state, federal and the executive branches of our government to pass legislation that will provide better quality cancer care for the millions of people affected by the disease. Cancer, its treatments, and the devastating affect on the lives it touches needs to be brought to the forefront of the American public.

Only then can we begin to find ways to make it the national priority that it needs to be. I am looking forward to taking what could have been a negative part of my life and using it to positively help others. I feel like I am in the best of company—Lance Armstrong, Jaclyn Smith, Fran Dresher, and countless other celebrities—and prominent political figures in today's society have all come out about how they or members of their families are coping with cancer.

If they can speak out about it, so can the millions of Americans also affected by this debilitating and chronic disease. Cancer is non-partisan and doesn't care who it strikes. We need to band together and strike back—finding a cure and making it as obsolete as some of the childhood diseases from decades ago. By becoming effective advocates, whether it is at the local, state, or federal level we can combine our voices and make ourselves heard. All of us who have been through cancer have a story, and each version is as unique as the person who experienced it.

A Note from the Author

This is my first attempt at writing a book. When I first started writing, it was to update an original story I had written about Dwayne's cancer for our support group in early 2007. After working on the update for over 3 weeks, and coming up with 13 pages, I stopped. It was my Admissions Advisor with Kaplan University, Xavier Napier, who convinced me that those pages were the framework of a good book—a short one to offer help to other people, while somehow providing additional income for us.

While searching on the internet one afternoon, I found a company and decided to submit the manuscript for review. I had the frame work in the 8 pages, and at the urging of many people, I sat down with my husband and began filling in all of the missing pieces with the events that happened to us both as we journeyed through cancer and it's side effects.

Well, those missing pieces are this book. Once I began to write, the words just seemed to flow, coming fast as I remembered all of the turmoil, depression and heartache that we endured throughout the journey we traveled.

But I feel very strongly that this story of survivorship needs to be told. All of the events depicted within these pages are true. I tried, with words, to paint as vivid a picture I could of what Dwayne felt, endured and came through on his way to survivorship.

Cancer is a life-changing illness that leaves its mark on each and every life it touches—whether it is that of the patient or his family, friends and caregiver. We are all battle weary and have the wounds to prove it.

Those who are going through the diagnosis and treatments often feel alone or abandoned and unsure of what to do or how they will survive all of this.

This is the story of one family's journey down that long and winding road that sometimes seemed as if it had no final destination, but was a rambling journey to nowhere. But through strength they didn't know they possessed, an unshakable Faith in God, and by leaning on each other each during every step of the way, they persevered.

It has been written in the hopes that it will help someone somewhere realize that they too can complete this unwanted journey. That they, too can make a difference in someone else's life as they share their stories, feelings, thoughts with someone whom they can help.

I would welcome any comments or suggestions you as the reader may have. It is important to me that you realize this was done as a way to reach out and bring awareness to this disease, and how it affects people in ways that, unless you've lived through it, you can't begin to imagine. I hope this will give you a small glimpse of what a person experiences.

The reason that I included the chapters concerning the power wheel chair and the fight with Medicare to obtain it, the loan, van, lift and ramp saga is because without those tools, we wouldn't be able to work as effective advocates for cancer issues due to my degenerative bone disease. It prevents me from being mobile without assistance

Please write to me at:

14375 Eheart Circle

Barboursville, VA 22923

OR at:

CntryAngel22923@aol.com

About the Author

Barbara was born in Goochland County, Virginia in 1960 and raised in a small rural farming community at the foot of the Blue Ridge Mountains — not far from Shenandoah National Park. This entire area of the Commonwealth is rich in history, and has many national tourist attractions, all within easy driving distance.

Her dad was a veteran of WWII and had been in the Normandy Invasion and the occupation of France. Her mother worked in a local textile factory, so she spent her days with aunt, uncle and dad on t he small farm.

Born with Cerebral Palsy, she underwent three separate orthopedic surgeries to lengthen her heel cords so she could walk, and wore corrective shoes and braces until age 18. She was shy and applied herself to her studies, and loved school. She excelled in spelling and English Composition throughout school.

Her general studies in high school were in the business curriculum and included Typing I and II, and Office Services I, II, III and IV, where she received numerous typing awards and earned the praises of all of her instructors. She was a member of the FBLA, and represented her school in the state finals of the Spelling Bee, where she placed second.

She worked in the main office, library, and cafeteria on the Work-Study program during her lunch and study hall periods; and as a senior she was employed by the University of Virginia Hospital as a CRT

Data entry clerk with the Medical Records Department, Statistics section.

After high school graduation she sought out assistance from the Virginia Department of Rehabilitative Services to continue her education at Woodrow Wilson Rehabilitation Center and studied the General Business Curriculum, where she received her certificate of completion in October of 1982.

Since graduation, she has held many positions in different fields including: Office Manager for UVa's Crisis Intervention Center, Acquisition Assistant at Jefferson-Madison Regional Library,

Housekeeper for two major companies: Redi-Maid and Butterfly Services, Inc., Cashier/Shift Manager for 7-11, Cook and cashier for Bodie-Noel, Inc., Home-Health Aid for three years, Inserter, machine operator and Pressman for a local newspaper, and Telemarketing Specialist for a major manufacturer.

In 1989 she was forced to apply for Social Security Disability due to chronic asthma that prevented her from working; after being on life-support on two different occasions.

Since then she has been involved with her church and their outreach ministry, spear-heading their toy lift participation for 3 years, and since my diagnosis with cancer, has really been active:

—in our support group

—baking for patients at the cancer center

—bringing a cancer advocacy program to the cancer center.

—working with a national cancer organization to push legislation in congress to benefit cancer patients.

She has become a voting member of C-PAC, the state Cancer Plan for our state.

She is more interested in working with this group to come up with viable state level plans that will benefit those receiving treatment and who have issues on various subjects pertaining to their survivorship.

LOOKING FORWARD

As we begin to go through January of 2008, there are a lot of unknowns. We also have a lot to look forward in this coming year and we are excited about the prospects of a lot of them.

I am beginning to get my bearings on this new job, and so far so good. However, if for some reason it doesn't work out, then I will just move on to something else, hopefully a job that is better in many respects. God has always provided for us when we didn't have a hope anywhere else, and we trust him to continue doing so.

Our work NCCS and cancer advocacy is going smoothly and we are enjoying what we do. There are the occasional trips to Washington, which in itself can be an adventure even before you get to Capitol Hill—and that's where it can really get exciting.

Barbara has decided to further her education and has enrolled as a student at Kaplan University online. She will be studying to become a medical transcriptionist, and in December, 2009 will have an Associate's Degree. Ok. She's excited and at the same time very apprehensive.

While she excelled in some subjects in her earlier years of school, there were some that caused major problems, including math—and algebra is a required class credit she has to have in order to graduate. Thankfully, one of the perks offered by the University is tutoring, which I'm sure she will take full advantage of.

I celebrated my 4th year anniversary of my diagnosis on January 24, 2008. I've made it through almost the entire 5 year watch program—THANK GOD! Of course, it hasn't been without incident.

I had a cancer scare a few months back when I went to an appointment with my Palliative Care Physician, Dr. Blackhall. She printed and gave me a copy of a cytology report from an earlier visit in Urology back in July of 2006. It floored both Barbara and myself and brought more than a few tears, many, many more.

The report showed abnormal cells in my bladder, indicative of some type or stage of bladder cancer, and I couldn't believe my eyes. Oh, God! Please! Don't tell me I have to go through another battle with this monster, was all I think as I walked back into the waiting room where Barbara was waiting for me.

Well, we cried and talked with Vikki. Barbara had Mark on the phone, trying to find some way to come to terms with the possibility, and he gave a person to contact whose husband was a survivor of bladder cancer, and had started a non-profit organization to help others.

I've had the lighted scope test done with negative results, praise God and will have to reschedule a CT scan that for one reason or another, I've had to miss twice already. Hopefully that will be negative as well. I'm trying hard to think positive about it. I've also been placed on Centroid, a medication to treat thyroid disease, since the level was extremely low. It is dangerous because it affects not only mood swings and metabolism (which is probably why I wasn't gaining weight) but can also cause damage to organs and tissues. I will take it for the rest of my life, which is no big deal after having defeated cancer. Since being on the medication, we've noticed improvements in every aspect for which I am very thankful.

We are looking forward our group meetings this year and being as active, if not more so than we were last year, and Barbara is assuming the role of newspaper editor, which she enjoys.

Mark and the staff at NCCS are working hard to find a date that suits everyone so that we can make a visit to the office in Silver Spring for a meeting with everyone. Barbara has talked to almost all of the key staff members, including the CEO and President, Ellen Stovall, among others. I think the only person she has yet to introduce herself to is the COO Michael Bergen, but I'm sure that will come in time.

We are both excited about finding a way to share this book with other patients and survivors who have been diagnosed and who have battled cancer. It is something that we want to share especially with those who have been recently diagnosed. They are shell shocked and wondering how in the world they will find the strength to get through all of the things they will have to face. It's not easy, but trust me it can be done. It takes willpower, grit and determination; and it will test your faith in everything you've ever known, but with a positive attitude you can make it…you too can become a SURVIVOR!!!!!!!!!!

God Bless!

9 781606 108468